T0200033

Dissociation

Culture, Mind, and Body

Dissociation

Culture, Mind, and Body

Edited by David Spiegel, M.D.

Department of Psychiatry and Behavioral Sciences
Stanford University School of Medicine
Stanford, California

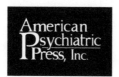

Washington, DC
London, England

Note: The authors have worked to ensure that all information in this book concerning drug dosages, schedules, and routes of administration is accurate as of the time of publication and consistent with standards set by the U.S. Food and Drug Administration and the general medical community. As medical research and practice advance, however, therapeutic standards may change. For this reason and because human and mechanical errors sometimes occur, we recommend that readers follow the advice of a physician who is directly involved in their care or the care of a member of their family.

Books published by the American Psychiatric Press, Inc., represent the views and opinions of the individual authors and do not necessarily represent the policies and opinions of the Press or the American Psychiatric Association.

Copyright © 1994 American Psychiatric Press, Inc.
ALL RIGHTS RESERVED
Manufactured in the United States of America on acid-free paper
97 96 95 94   4 3 2 1
First Edition

American Psychiatric Press, Inc.
1400 K Street, N.W., Washington, DC   20005

Library of Congress Cataloging-in-Publication Data
Dissociation : culture, mind, and body / [edited by] David Spiegel. —
   1st ed.
      p. cm.
   Includes bibliographical references and index.
   ISBN 0-88048-557-4
   1. Dissociation (Psychology) 2. Dissociative disorders.
3. Mental healing. 4. Dissociation (Psychology)—Social aspects.
I. Spiegel, David, 1945–   .
   [DNLM: 1. Dissociative Disorders. 2. Mental Healing.
3. Consciousness.   WM 173.6 D613 1994]
RC553.D5D55   1994
616.85′23—dc20
DNLM/DLC
for Library of Congress   93-47478
                                                                    CIP

British Library Cataloguing in Publication Data
A CIP record is available from the British Library.

Contents

Section I:
Dissociation: The Phenomenon

Section II:
Measuring Dissociation

Section III:
Culture and Dissociation

Section IV:
Dissociation: Mind and Body

Contributors

Kenneth S. Bowers, Ph.D.
Department of Psychology, University of Waterloo, Waterloo, Ontario, Canada

Eve B. Carlson, Ph.D.
Department of Psychology, Beloit College, Beloit, Wisconsin

Matthew Hugh Erdelyi, Ph.D.
Department of Psychology, Brooklyn College, and the Graduate School of The City University of New York, Brooklyn, New York

Laurence J. Kirmayer, M.D., F.R.C.P.C.
Division of Social and Transcultural Psychiatry, Department of Psychiatry, McGill University, and Institute of Community and Family Psychiatry, Sir M.B. Davis—Jewish General Hospital, Montreal, Quebec, Canada

Roberto Lewis-Fernández, M.D.
Department of Social Medicine, Harvard Medical School, Boston, Massachusetts, and Latino Mental Health Clinic, The Cambridge Hospital, Department of Psychiatry, Cambridge, Massachusetts

Colin A. Ross, M.D.
Dissociative Disorders Unit, Charter Hospital of Dallas, Plano, Texas

David Spiegel, M.D.
Department of Psychiatry and Behavioral Sciences, Stanford University School of Medicine, Stanford, California

Marlene Steinberg, M.D.
Yale University School of Medicine, New Haven, Connecticut

Eric Vermutten, M.D.
Department of Psychiatry and Behavioral Sciences, Stanford University School of Medicine, Stanford, California

Introduction

"There is no such entity as consciousness: we are from moment to moment differently conscious."

—Hughlings Jackson, 1931[1]

Dissociation, the compartmentalization of experience, identity, memory, perception, and motor function, challenges many comfortable assumptions. Dissociative phenomena are often stark, extreme, and vivid. Memory for an entire period of time during which one was conscious seems lost. Identities shift between apparent opposites. Pain is ignored. Trauma victims transform the experience and report floating above their injured bodies. Are these arcane, dramatic, or even staged events, or does dissociation underlie some fundamental aspect of mental organization? Is it merely the product of a troubled mind, or a key to understanding the structure of consciousness and the mind-body relationship? Is dissociation normal and the everyday perception of mental unity the delusion?

These are hard questions, but dissociative phenomena are so interesting that they are being asked and answered. Why is it that healing ceremonies around the world seem to involve alterations in consciousness with dissociative features? It has been observed in the anthropological literature that there are three basic parts to healing rituals. First, the person becomes aware of being in a state of disease and seeks help from a healer of some kind. Second, he or she goes to the healer and one or both enter an altered state of consciousness, sometimes with somatic conversion symptoms, sometimes becoming quiet and hyporesponsive. Battle is done with the illness, and the patient's understanding of the illness and of what effect it will have upon him or her is altered. Third, the patient leaves the healing

---

[1] Cited in Levinson B: "The States of Awareness in Anaesthesia in 1965," in *Memory and Awareness in Anaesthesia*. Edited by Bonke B, Fitch W, Millar K. Amsterdam, Swets & Zeitlinger, 1990, pp 11–18.

ceremony with some new perspective about the disease and, hopefully, with an improvement in symptoms. This process occurs even in high-tech Western medicine, although the cultural rituals surrounding the mental transformations are quite different. Dissociative changes in mental state have been associated with changed cognition and somatic function for millennia. Highly hypnotizable individuals seem uniquely capable of altering somatic function using dissociative mechanisms. Dissociation may well have something to teach us about the association between mind and body.

Scientific research about the mind-body problem in the twentieth century has been single-mindedly deterministic. We have taken the Aristotelian reductionist approach, which holds that mind is the product of its biology but does not influence it. To understand the mind-body problem, this line of thought holds, one must understand the body and the brain. Tremendous advances have been made in understanding brain neurochemistry through the study of neurotransmitters, psychopharmacology, brain imaging, and molecular genetics. Nonetheless, our advancing computational technology allows us to attack, with relative precision, problems of greater complexity and provides the possibility of examining the mind and brain in interaction with the body. This means treating the whole as greater than the sum of its parts.

Interest in the role of dissociative and hypnotic phenomena as mediators of the mind-body relationship led the John D. and Catherine T. MacArthur Foundation to convene a network of investigators to develop a collaborative research agenda. The problem posed to us by board member and Nobel Prize-winning physicist Murray Gell-Mann was, "Figure out how hypnosis cures warts." He saw that truly understanding this odd but well-replicated observation could lead to a major advance in appreciating the interaction between mind and body. How does a change in mental state (hypnosis) coupled with content directed at eliminating warts (tingling, numbness, picturing them shrivel and drop off) result in this actually happening on the body in a substantial portion of cases?

Over 4 years, a research group was assembled, and it developed a plan of exploration of this and related phenomena. As of this time, it consists of J. Allan Hobson, M.D., sleep researcher at Harvard University; Steven Kosslyn, Ph.D., an experimental psychologist at Harvard interested in the brain mechanisms underlying imagery; Kenneth Hugdahl, Ph.D., an experimental neuropsychologist from the University of Bergen in Norway with special interests in brain laterality; Arthur Kleinman, M.D., Ph.D., a Harvard psychiatrist and anthropologist; Robert Rose, M.D., a psychiatrist at the MacArthur

Introduction

Foundation and Rush Medical School with expertise in the psychoendo-
crinology of stress; Mardi Horowitz, M.D., a research psychoanalyst at the
University of California in San Francisco; and myself from Stanford, a research psychiatrist with interests in hypnosis, dissociation, and psychosocial
effects on cancer progression.

Our group believed that a conference on dissociative phenomena span-
ning culture, mind, and body would facilitate our work. This belief led to
a conference at the Center for Advanced Study in the Behavioral Sciences
in Stanford, California, on October 17–19, 1991, sponsored by the Research
Network on Mind-Body Interactions of the John D. and Catherine T. Mac-
Arthur Foundation. Experts in cognitive psychology, dissociation, cultural
anthropology, hypnosis, and psychophysiology convened to examine these
issues. What follows are selected, carefully written papers given at the conference and then extensively revised. They thus reflect the best thinking of
the authors in response to interaction with other experts from diverse fields.
They represent a sympathetic but critical examination of dissociation from
social, cognitive, and neurophysiological perspectives and shed important
light on the contribution of the phenomena to our understanding of culture,
mind, and body.

Matthew Erdelyi, Ph.D., a noted memory researcher and integrator of
cognitive and psychodynamic theory (Erdelyi 1985), first intrigues us with
a historical overview of the resiliency of the concept of dissociation. He
notes that one can find traces of the idea at least as far back as the ancient
Greek philosophers and that even though it may be abandoned (or dissociated) for long periods of our cultural history, it keeps reappearing, for
good reason. He describes it as presenting a challenge to our comfortable
Western assumption of mental unity and individual identity. He makes the
bold and well-defended claim that indeed dissociation is a necessary part
of complex mental functioning and may subsume the notion of the unconscious itself. He then presents experimental evidence from perception and
memory research to illustrate that dissociation is a ubiquitous, necessary,
and normal mental structure.

Kenneth Bowers, Ph.D., a highly regarded cognitive psychologist, provides a novel view of the phenomena underlying hypnosis, a form of structured dissociation coupled with highly focused attention and extreme
sensitivity to social cues. He reviews data suggesting that hypnotic reduction of pain, for example, may proceed via two rather different pathways.
On the one hand, some highly hypnotizable individuals achieve analgesia
by focusing on and becoming absorbed in an image that carries with it an

intense experience of relief—putting the injured hand into a bucket of ice chips, for example. In hypnosis, the image is so vivid that it is felt as well as thought of, and it produces substantial analgesia. But Dr. Bowers notes that some hypnotized individuals do just as well or better by simply turning off sensation in the injured hand and thinking about something else, as though they were tapping some automatic subroutine. This use of hypnosis seems to provide access to low-level control systems that are not usually accessed in consciousness.

Eve B. Carlson, Ph.D., who is the first author of the most widely used scale of dissociation, The Dissociative Experiences Scale (DES), summarizes its reliability, validity, factor structure, and relationship to hypnotizability. The three main factors include amnesia, absorption, and depersonalization and derealization.

Dr. Carlson notes that certain somatic disorders have been found to be associated with higher scores on the DES. These include the luteal phase of premenstrual syndrome and bulimia, suggesting a possible interactive effect. Although she emphasizes that the endocrine and eating disorders may underlie dissociative symptomatology, there may also be a dissociative component to the emotional disturbance. Some bulimic patients, for example, report feeling in a dissociative state when engaged in their compulsive eating behavior (Pettinati 1985). She notes that there is little evidence suggesting a link between seizure disorders and dissociation but does find several studies that show that patients with a history of physical and sexual abuse obtain substantially higher scores on the DES. In addition, such patients show a higher ability to tolerate pain in the laboratory. Thus this body of research suggests that dissociation may be elicited by, and may in turn represent an adaptation to, somatic distress, especially that involving pain, endocrine function, and eating behavior.

Interestingly, disorders of the nervous system, which seem to be a prime candidate, have in recent research not been shown to be associated with dissociative symptoms. However, the issue of the co-occurrence of certain kinds of seizure disorders, such as complex partial seizures, and dissociative symptoms needs further exploration (Spiegel 1991). It may well be that there is a dissociative syndrome associated with certain kinds of temporal lobe epilepsy that is phenomenologically similar to classical dissociative disorders but historically distinct. That is, these individuals may have dissociative amnesia, fugue, depersonalization, derealization, and other symptoms but may not have the history of sexual and physical trauma that is so typical of dissociative disorder patients. Thus it is unlikely that one explains the other, but it may well be that there are certain common mechanisms. In any event, the data reviewed in this chapter suggest that certain endocrine and gastrointestinal disorders are associated with higher prevalence of dissociative symptoms.

Dissociation can be measured as a normal phenomenon, as Dr. Carlson has done it, potentially occurring throughout the population. On the other hand, dissociative disorders are florid but rarer illnesses that occur among psychiatric patients. They can be understood as more extreme and uncontrolled eruptions of these normal phenomena, often elicited in the face of traumatic stress.

Marlene Steinberg, M.D., a Yale psychiatrist, has developed the Structured Clinical Interview for DSM-IV Dissociative Disorders (SCID-D). It provides a reliable and valid means of establishing the presence or absence of such disorders. She describes the major components of these disorders as affecting memory, identity, and perception of the body and the surrounding environment. Thus dissociative phenomena may underlie both the organization and the pathological disorganization of mental and physical function.

Laurence Kirmayer, M.D., F.R.C.P.C., a psychiatrist and expert on cross-cultural psychiatry and somatization, describes cultural influences on the manifestations of dissociation. Social forces may serve to make the most of underlying hypnotic and dissociative abilities. Trance dancing in Bali is often taught "body-up," the teacher moving the student's compliant body rather than explaining or demonstrating the movements. He notes that dissociative phenomena in the West often involve disruptions of identity, such as dissociative identity disorder (formerly called multiple personality disorder). This may underscore the Western preoccupation with the individual and illustrate that identity is in many ways a nonunitary social construct, an idea more congenial in the Orient.

Roberto Lewis-Fernández, M.D., a research fellow and psychiatrist at Harvard, pursues this theme in detail, examining the effect of cultural differences on the configuration of two dissociative disorders: Puerto Rican *ataque de nervios* and Indian "possession syndrome."

Dr. Lewis-Fernández notes that there are both important commonalities and differences in the way dissociative phenomena emerge across cultures. Both seem to afflict disadvantaged individuals in their cultures, those of lower socioeconomic status with some history of life disadvantage or trauma, and family disruptions such as divorce or death, and yet there are important differences. Possession syndrome involves the transformation of identity. The possessed individual enters a trance-like state and feels that his or her personal identity is superseded by that of an invading, outside force. On the other hand, patients with *ataque de nervios* suffer a variety of experiential and somatic changes and worry about them but show no disruption in their sense of personal identity. Dr. Lewis-Fernández attributes this difference in part to social definitions of identity and preoccupations with spirituality. The very malleability of individuals prone to dissociation can make them a kind of cultural barometer, prone to exhibit symptoms along cultural fault lines that may reflect either important points of cultural stress, contradiction or conflict, or areas of considerable cultural attention and importance.

In "Dissociation and Physical Illness," Colin Ross, M.D., provides a theoretical model in which a history of physical and sexual abuse produces the mental effect of dissociation and the physical effect of somatization. Thus these two co-occur but are not seen as causing one another. Dr. Ross refers to evidence that patients with extreme dissociative disorders, such as dissociative identity, show unusual somatic symptoms as well. He postulates a more generic model in which somatic disorders involving genitourinary functioning are natural consequences of sexual abuse. In addition, he provides evidence from his own research that disorders of the gastrointestinal tract, such as irritable bowel syndrome, are associated with a history of trauma. This is interesting in view of Whorewell's (1984) controlled study showing that hypnosis can be effective in treating irritable bowel syndrome. Coupled with Dr. Carlson's finding of a link between dissociation and luteal phase and eating disorders, it may be that disruption of certain somatic systems such as the gastrointestinal and endocrine system may be associated with a greater use of dissociative defenses.

Dr. Ross also summarizes his Dissociative Disorders Interview Schedule designed to yield a DSM-III-R diagnosis and examines its relationship to measures of somatization. He calls for further research on the relationship between dissociation and somatization.

In our article, "Physiological Correlates of Hypnosis and Dissociation," I and Eric Vermutten, M.D., review data on mind-brain and mind-body control evidenced during hypnotic and dissociative phenomena. Highly hypnotizable individuals seem to have an unusual capacity to control both mental functions, such as perception, memory, and attention, and somatic functions, especially in certain systems available to awareness (i.e., the gastrointestinal system, nervous systems involving motor function, and the skin). The changes highly hypnotizable people can produce are disciplined and reversible. They seem to reflect not so much being in or out of the trance state, per se, as they do the task undertaken within the trance state. For example, in highly hypnotizable individuals taught to obstruct perception of a stimulus using hypnotic hallucination, changes can be observed in brain electrophysiological response to those stimuli. Highly hypnotizable individuals can learn to increase or decrease the flow of gastric acid, the presence of irritable bowel symptoms, and pain. Thus hypnosis and the less structured dissociative phenomena seem to provide enhanced access to control systems that interconnect mind and body. By demonstrating the limits of our ability to modulate these control systems, we may learn more not only about how mind and body interact but how cultural, social, and mental phenomena may adversely or therapeutically influence the health of the body.

In this book you will find not so much complete agreement as a thoughtful examination of intersecting issues and, hopefully, a useful integration of the related cultural, mental, and physical aspects of dissociation.

REFERENCES

Erdelyi MH: Psychoanalysis: Freud's Cognitive Psychology. New York, WH Freeman, 1985

Pettinati HM, Horne RL, Staats JM: Hypnotizability in patients with anorexia nervosa and bulimia. Arch Gen Psychiatry 42:1014–1016, 1985

Spiegel D: Neurophysiological correlates of hypnosis and dissociation. Journal of Neuropsychiatry 3:440–445, 1991

Whorewell PJ, Prior A, Faragher EB: Controlled trial of hypnotherapy in the treatment of severe refractory irritable bowel syndrome. Lancet 1:1232–1234, 1984

Section I

Dissociation: The Phenomenon

CHAPTER 1

Dissociation, Defense, and the Unconscious

Matthew Hugh Erdelyi, Ph.D.

D issociationism designates a theoretical commitment to the notion that integrated systems such as the self are made up of subsystems that may become—or may even normally be—relatively disconnected in terms of information exchange or mutual control. I will direct my remarks in this opening chapter to some basic questions about dissociationism, such as, Why dissociationism? Why is it still around? How does it fit into modern cognitive psychology?

There is a straightforward generic answer: Dissociationism has been around, persists, is ingrained in cognitive psychology, and will continue to be around because it is a fundamental reality of psychology, indeed of any complex living system. Dissociationism will always be with us (I predict), though it is possible that it will be absorbed into some other conceptual framework. But I doubt it. On the contrary, I believe dissociationism will absorb other concepts—the unconscious, for example—as I shall try to show in the latter part of this chapter.

This chapter is divided into two main sections, one broad brushed, the other fine grained. The first is a general theoretical and historical overview of dissociationism that is undergirded by a general systems framework. The second is a demonstration section. It is a technical application of dissociationism to a classic construct of psychology—clinical and cognitive—

This work was supported by Grants 6-67442, 6-68464, and 6-61291 from The City University of New York PSC-CUNY Research Award Program.

the *unconscious,* in which it is shown that two types of dissociation define and subsume all the manifold expressions of the unconscious. The unconscious is thus shown to be a derivative concept of the bedrock notion of dissociation.

GENERAL OVERVIEW OF THE HISTORY AND THEORY OF DISSOCIATION

Dissociation and Polypsychism

Dissociationism in the history of dynamic psychology arises from the breakdown of an illusion—or, at least, what many consider to be an illusion—*the illusion of the unity of self.* Presently, I will backtrack a bit and argue, in what may appear to skirt primary process logic, that the unity of self is an illusion and is not an illusion—p and not-p. But for the present I will adopt the illusion hypothesis: The unitary *self* is an illusion.

Because of space constraints—and my ignorance—I will not attempt to delve into ancient traditions, such as Hindu and Buddhist thinking, which is so riveted on the notion of *maya* (illusion), especially in matters involving the self, and will begin by asserting that the nonunity of self has a long-standing history in Western thinking. This is the tradition of *polypsychism,* the notion that the self—the *I,* the *ego*—is made up of many subsystems (Ellenberger 1970).

One might begin with Plato who, in clear anticipation of Freud's ego-superego-id triad of self, pointed (in *The Republic,* for example) to reason, shame, and "the beast" within us. But to cut through two millennia of philosophic underbrush, we might, with Ellenberger (1970), go back to St. Augustine's *Confessions.* St. Augustine was perplexed. As a Christian he felt that he was a new man, and yet in his dreams his pagan self frequently emerged. He wondered about the dreamer's moral responsibility for the dream personality. And so we have in St. Augustine the notion of two personalities inhabiting one person.

We humans have a developmental proclivity in counting: First, 1; then, 2; finally, many. The polypsychist view, which supersedes the self-as-one notion, tends to start as a dualism—in which case it may be designated *dipsychism* (Ellenberger 1970, pp. 143–144).

Many *fin de siècle* thinkers embraced a dipsychist view. Binet (1889–

1890) developed the notion in his book, *On Double Consciousness,* to account for cases of "dual personality" (Ellenberger 1970, pp. 143–144; Hilgard 1977, p. 4). Max Dessoir (1890/1986) elaborated a similar theme in his book, *Das Dopple-Ich (The Double-Ego;* Ellenberger 1970, p. 145; Hilgard 1977, p. 4), contrasting "upper-consciousness" with "under-consciousness," the latter corresponding to the consciousness of dreams and the hypnotic state. The American gynecologist A. F. A. King thought that the key to the riddle was the clash between "two departments of physiological government" in the individual: 1) the department of self-preservation and 2) the department of reproduction (Ellenberger 1970, pp. 143–144). Pierre Janet, in *Psychological Automatism* (1889), also espoused a dipsychist view: In certain individuals—pathological cases—a "dissociation" (*désagrégation*) of personality (ego) occurs. Part of the personality splits off to become an autonomous subconscious subpersonality. As Hilgard (1977, p. 6) noted, Morton Prince (1906), in his *The Dissociation of Personality,* prefers *coconscious* to *subconscious* because each different subsystem might be invested with consciousness. The possible consciousness of alternate subsystems should not, however, be regarded as a difficulty for the concept of the unconscious (see Erdelyi 1985) because, from the standpoint of a reference subsystem, the information in other subsystems that it cannot access is legitimately unconscious/subconscious to it, regardless of whether the information is or is not conscious to the other subsystems.

It is not necessary, of course, to restrict oneself to a dualistic dissociation. One may pull out the stops and adopt *polypsychism,* a term coined (according to Ellenberger 1970, pp. 146 ff) by Durand (de Gros), who posited a system involving an "ego-in-chief" and "a legion of subegos" (each with its own consciousness!). He assumed, like so many in the dynamic psychology tradition, that in hypnosis the ego-in-chief is pushed aside and direct access to some of the subegos is achieved.

Sigmund Freud, of course, advanced his own brand of polypsychism. In 1923 he posited two subsystems of personality (the ego and the id) but by 1933 was up to three subsystems, the id, the ego, and the superego. More noteworthy than his counting to three is Freud's *dynamic* conception of mental dissociation, which distinguishes him from the likes of Janet, and to which I shall soon turn.

Perhaps one of the most central figures of polypsychism and dissociationism, curiously neglected by modern psychology, is Carl Gustav Jung, who was influenced by both Janet (he had taken a course of his) and Freud. In his book *Analytical Psychology* (1935/1968), which to a surprising extent is based on experimental studies (of doubtful methodology, however), he states: "The so-called unity of consciousness is an illusion . . . . We like to think that we are one; but we are not, most decidedly not" (p. 81). (The statement echoes Janet's: "There are crowds of things which operate within ourselves without our will" [Ellenberger 1970, p. 370].)

Jung strikingly anticipates contemporary modularity theorists (e.g., Fodor 1983; Gazzaniga 1985) and schemata/states theorists (e.g., Horowitz 1991). For Jung, the module or schema is the *Vorstellungskomplex,* an emotionally charged complex of representations—*complex,* for short: "Complexes are autonomous groups of associations that have a tendency to move by themselves, to live their own life apart from our intentions . . . . This idea explains a lot" (Jung 1935/1968, p. 81). "[C]omplexes . . . are fragmentary personalities" (p. 82). (I oversimplify matters by bypassing Jung's deeper strata of substructures, the *archetypes.*)

Very much in the tradition of Binet and Janet, Jung (1935/1968) viewed the manifestation of the subpersonalities as constituting *hysteria* or, more generally, *neurosis:* "A neurosis is a dissociation of personality due to the existence of complexes" (p. 188).

Jung also incorporated Herbartian and Freudian dynamics into his scheme: Complexes, in the Herbartian mold, struggle for dominance; the complex that is dominant at t_1 is the "ego . . . one's subjective self." But another complex may displace the previous complex at t_2, hence a new "personality." Also, Freud's *defense* concept is incorporated in that a dominant complex may defensively fend off an emotionally unacceptable complex.

It is difficult not to discern echoes of Jung in modern modularity theories.

Michael Gazzaniga (1985), in *The Social Brain,* presents a modularistic neuroscience perspective. He sees some links to Freud—the unconscious is associated with the activity of "nonverbal mental modules," and it is suggested at one point that "Freud in his own way presaged much of modern cognitive psychology" (p. 117)—Gazzaniga nevertheless sounds more like Jung:

> I think this notion of linear unified conscious experience is dead wrong. In contrast, I argue that the human brain has a modular-type organization . . . . The brain is organized into relatively independent functioning units (p. 4). . . . hundreds of them or maybe even thousands . . . these modules can usually express themselves only through real action, not through ver-

bal communication. Most of these systems . . . can remember events, store affective reactions to these events, and respond to stimuli associated with a particular memory. (p. 77)

Modularity, Gazzaniga emphasizes, necessarily implies the occurrence of "striking dissociations" (p. 109). This essentially has been my point too: Polypsychism and dissociationism are necessarily linked, dissociation being the necessary consequence—and indicator—of polypsychism.

Now a few words on my own spin on the theme:

1. Yes, the self is made up of modules/complexes/whatevers.
2. But, the modules are made up of modules themselves.
3. The self itself is a module (e.g., in the family system, as family systems theory emphasizes).
4. A higher-order module (e.g., the family) is in turn a module of a still larger social system.

My stance, then, is a *general systems theory* stance (e.g., Koestler 1967; Miller 1978; von Bertalanffy 1968): All systems are simultaneously sub- and suprasystems; what is a *legitimate system* at one level is a *subsystem* at another level and a *suprasystem* at still a different level. And so, the unity of the self can, depending on one's system vantage point, be real or illusory.

Subjectively, most of us have a compelling sense of unified self; the self does not seem to us usually to be an illusory entity: *I* was asked to write this; *I* accepted; *I* am writing. Indeed, if we did not have a compelling sense of a unitary self, dissociationism would make little sense. Suppose the following: Mary loves John but Susan hates him. This is not a dissociation unless Mary and Susan are subpersonalities of, in some sense, a single individual. At some level then, even if only subjectively, there must be a unit for dissociation to arise. Dissociation represents some discrepant manifestation of a system's subsystems; both the system and its subsystems are *sine qua nons* of dissociation. What is striking about dissociation is that it jars us, unawares, from one system level to another. The subsystem's discrepant manifestations capture our attention, and what we were conceiving of as a system we suddenly see, in Necker-cube fashion, as subsystems, and the previous system level now appears illusory.

When the subsystems of the *I* are collaborating harmoniously, it is easy to forget that the *I* is made up of subsystems, though there is never pure harmony and there are always ongoing dissociations that by habit we ignore

7

(shifts in mood, change of states as in dreams, etc.). In cases of extreme disharmony of the *I* system, the illusion of self becomes problematic: The patient says he (or she) is happy, but he complains that he wakes up early and can't fall back asleep; he sighs a lot; he loses weight markedly. Is he happy or depressed—or both? The split-brain patient is the most dramatic example.

When the self-system is in disharmony, as in a civil war, the subsystems become more obvious or salient. Pushed far enough, the system no longer seems tenable (e.g., the former Soviet Union).

The political/sociological analogy is a powerful one. General systems theory holds that homologous laws may be discovered across systems levels. So the analogies may not be idle figures of speech; one level of system may reasonably "model" other levels of systems. There may thus be good reasons for the frequent intertwining of sociological, psychological, and physiological metaphors, as in the *nerves of government* (Deutsch 1966); the *social brain* (Gazzaniga 1985); *parliament of instincts* (Lorenz 1966); *departments of physiological government* (A. F. A. King, see previous comments); *censorship, economic model, repression/suppression,* and so on (see Freud sources discussed in Erdelyi 1985); and *a war of nerves* (Hobson 1988).

Just as with the self, dissociations exist at subsystems levels. In the limbic system, for example, the amygdala is a "hawk" urging the hypothalamus "executive" (in the ventromedial nucleus) to aggress, while the septum, the "dove," counsels calm and peace. Even at the synaptic level the theme unfolds, with some neurotransmitters in the synaptic cleft urging "GO!" but other neurotransmitters countering "NO!" So there are conflicts/discrepancies/contradictions at all systems levels—above the self, below the self, and at the level of the self.

The basic point then is that the systems view, however one frames it (polypsychism, modularity, states of mind, etc.), necessarily yields *dissociations*—contradictory contents or controls. These dissociations may be relatively subtle when the system is in harmony, striking when the system is stressed or damaged (e.g., hysteria, brain damage, civil war).

Janetian and Freudian Dissociations

In the history of psychology, two types of dissociations have been described, though not always under the name *dissociation*. Ernest Hilgard (1977, p. 10), for example, under the heading "The Decline of Dissociation," noted that the concept of dissociation waned for some decades because psychoanalytic psychology, which was for a while so popular, "substituted repression for dissociation." Indeed, one type of dissociationism was supplanted. However, *dissociationism* itself was not abandoned or absorbed, but rather a dissociationism different from Janet's was pursued. This would have been a positive development if the gain of the new had not resulted in the loss of the old.

Janetian dissociationism is a deficit phenomenon. Insufficiency of binding energy, caused by hereditary factors, life stresses, or traumas, or an interaction among them, results in a splitting off of personality clusters from the *ego,* the core personality. The split-off clusters or fragments constitute minipersonalities or, if they cohere, an alternate personality.

Freudian dissociation is an active defense phenomenon. Subsystems of ideas/wishes/thoughts/memories that threaten the integrity of the overall system (as judged by a judging subsystem, Freud's *ego*) are forcibly suppressed/repressed/inhibited/dissociated/split off, and so on:

> According to the theory of Janet . . . the splitting of consciousness is a primary feature of the mental change in hysteria. It is based on an innate weakness of the capacity for psychical synthesis. (Freud 1894/1962, p. 46)
>
> I repeatedly succeeded in demonstrating that the splitting of the contents of consciousness is the consequence of a voluntary act on the part of the patient; that is to say, it is instituted by an effort of will, the motive of which is discernible. (Freud 1894/1963, p. 69)

Although I disagree with Janet on some points (e.g., the assumption that dissociation and therefore the subconscious are restricted to psychopathological cases, even if I too stress that pathology in systems makes dissociation salient), I side with him as against Freud in two respects: 1) I agree with Janet's inclusive stance; he accepted Freud's defensive dissociation as a legitimate type of dissociation along with his own. 2) I also agree with Janet's conception of the subconscious/unconscious as "*une façon de parler*" (which Freud excoriated as scientific wishy-washiness, or worse).

With regard to the first issue—whether dissociations arise from *insufficiency* or *defense*—the debate, ironically, is reemerging within psychoanalysis without psychoanalysts realizing that they are revisiting the Janet-Freud cleavage (e.g., is *alexithymia* [Nemiah 1984] an incapacity to feel or express emotions, fantasy, imagery, or a defense against such feelings and experiences?).

The *defense-deficiency* controversy need not exist; both types of dissociation are operative.

In memory, for example, not thinking about some subject matter—whether because of defense or attentional neglect—should produce amnesia. Ebbinghaus (1885/1964) produced the first laboratory demonstration of this fact, showing that lists of memorized nonsense syllables that were deliberately not thought of undergo systematic forgetting over time. As I have emphasized (see Erdelyi 1990, 1993), the Ebbinghaus effect—forgetting—should automatically kick in regardless of the reason for the attentional neglect. This is something neither psychoanalysts nor cognitive psychologists have sufficiently considered. Also often ignored by cognitive psychologists is the fate of the forgotten, which is typically (and quite implicitly) assumed to be permanently lost, when in fact, as has been repeatedly shown experimentally, the forgotten can be partly recovered through retrieval effort (i.e., thinking; for further discussion, see Erdelyi 1990, 1993; Erdelyi and Becker 1974; Erdelyi and Kleinbard 1978; Roediger and Thorpe 1978; Payne 1987).

Further, the classic Ebbinghaus effect is not general (see Erdelyi 1990, 1993; M. H. Erdelyi, unpublished observations, 1994; Erdelyi and Kleinbard 1978). In fact, it is now a common view that, like the self, memory itself is not unitary and is therefore bound to yield striking dissociations under some circumstances. Such dissociations have been one of the breathless stories of cognitive psychology over the past decade or two (e.g., Bornstein and Pittman 1992; Lewandowsky et al. 1989; Parkin 1987; Singer 1990; Uleman and Bargh 1989).

To the extent that memory is not unitary, repression (not thinking/retrieval inhibition) need not have unitary effects. As I have suggested (Erdelyi 1990, 1993), what repression may do is to knock out certain aspects of memory (e.g., declarative) while sparing other memory systems (e.g., procedural memories).

The resulting dissociations in memory give a slightly different slant to Breuer and Freud's (1895/1955) classic formula, "hysterics suffer mainly from reminiscences" (p. 7), than to Freud's *conversion* notion. It is not that repressed memories are converted into symptoms (e.g., body memories) but that in the absence of conscious recollection—because of amnesia for declarative memories resulting from repression—the sequelae of traumas/conflicts persist in procedural formats, much to the puzzle of the patient. Thus my alternative to Freud's conversion hypothesis is that repression knocks out declarative memory (or certain types of modules/

complexes) but does not affect procedural memory (or other types of modules/complexes; Erdelyi 1990, 1993).

I have yet to find a reference to dreams in the modern memory literature. What kinds of memories do dreams represent? Procedural? Declarative? Both? If they in fact, as Freud strongly suggests, contain a substantial procedural component (dreams are *plastic-word representations, dramatizations)*, then, from the memory standpoint, dreams could after all be a royal road to the unconscious.

The declarative-procedural distinction is almost surely an oversimplification (remember: 1, 2, many). Therefore, though it is easier to speak in terms of dualities, what I really have in mind is that repression has differential effects on different modules/complexes. Nonunitary memory should yield nonunitary effects (i.e., dissociations).

With regard to the second issue, Janet's claim that the subconscious was only *une façon de parler*, Freud objected because the stance seemed to retreat from a full-fledged espousal of the reality of the unconscious. The unconscious became a construction, a story, a conceptual whimsy and ceased being, as bedrock nineteenth century science would have it, a true, palpable, no-nonsense entity. But this battle has been won and lost in twentieth century physics. Everyday notions like *force, time, electricity* are indeed intellectual constructions, and it is not the personal experience of the layperson (e.g., of gravity) but the mathematical formalizations that truly define what is aptly termed a *construct* (see Erdelyi 1985). Thus it is with the unconscious. It is not a place, a thing, or even a process. It is a construct—a construction, a manner of speaking or thinking, a story—that from the scientific standpoint must be defined formally. It is precisely such a formalization, in terms of dissociation, that I now wish to present. This formalization is rendered in the mathematics of inequalities (ordinal scales).

THE DISSOCIATION AND RECOVERY PARADIGMS OF THE UNCONSCIOUS

An unruly crowd of phenomena—from subception, autonomic conditioning, learning without awareness, and blindsight to dreams, symptoms, hypnosis, and multiple personality—have been advanced as empirical warrantors of the unconscious. Do these, in fact, provide the requisite evidence? And if so, need they be considered one by one to evaluate the status of the unconscious, or can some underlying logic to the evidence be discovered to cut through its surface diversity? I (Erdelyi 1985) have proposed that two logical structures, the *dissociation* and the *recovery* paradigms, can encompass all the phenomena legitimately advanced in support of the unconscious.

The Dissociation Paradigm of the Unconscious

The first of these, the dissociation paradigm, is by far the most widely employed in contemporary psychology. It is based on the discrepancy of information conveyed by two concurrent indicators of information: one, α, an indicator of information accessible to consciousness, and the other, ε, a more general indicator of information availability, such that $\varepsilon > \alpha$ (see Erdelyi 1985, 1986; Eriksen 1958; Goldiamond 1958; Reingold and Merikle 1988). (Indicators must be resorted to because mental contents cannot be observed directly.) The logic of the dissociation paradigm is that if the accessibility indicator, α (commonly linked these days with *explicit* or *direct* measures), conveys less information than another indicator, ε (e.g., an *indirect* or *implicit* measure), this necessarily means that more information is available than accessible to consciousness (i.e., there exists unconscious information).

In the unconscious perception (*subception*) literature, a constrained version of the dissociation paradigm has been traditionally employed, one in which the accessibility indicator, α, is set at zero. Thus $\varepsilon > \alpha \mid \alpha = 0$. In this constrained version, the thematic conundrum has been the validity of the null measure: Just because the measure is null, is accessibility necessarily null? For example, in the famous perceptual defense study of McGinnies (1949), in which it was shown that on preidentification threshold trials ($\alpha = 0$) tachistoscopic taboo stimuli were nevertheless discriminated by GSRs ($\varepsilon > 0$), the question immediately arose whether the effect was merely a response suppression artifact in which the subject withheld reporting embarrassing percepts of which he or she was unsure (see Erdelyi 1974). This would constitute discrimination without verbal response (a response dissociation) rather than discrimination without conscious perception (a mental dissociation). The reason that the Kunst-Wilson and Zajonc (KWZ) effect (Kunst-Wilson and Zajonc 1980) has stirred so much interest is that the accessibility measure used, recognition, credibly reflects chance-level performance ($\alpha = 0$), whereas the availability measure, preference, is above chance level ($\varepsilon > 0$).

Subception effects based on chance-level performance of α (e.g., Erdelyi's [1986] *absolute subliminality;* Merikle and Cheesman's [1986] *objective threshold*) are considered the most stringent demonstration of unconscious perception/memory and are judged by some to be improbable (Macmillan 1986) or, even, "impossible" (Bowers 1984). Merikle and Cheesman's subjective threshold, on the other hand, seems essentially to correspond to the subject's *decision criterion.* Subcriterion perception has never been in doubt—indeed, it has been traditionally treated as an artifact in the subliminal perception literature—and its existence is a basic premise of signal detection theory (see Erdelyi 1993).

It is in the nature of the laboratory to simplify conditions. In real-life situations, as in the clinic, it is unusual to rely on merely two indicators. More typically, two sets of indicators, one associated with availability, [ε], and the other with accessibility, [α], are contrasted. The dissociation paradigm with such "complex" indicators (Erdelyi 1985) is realized when [ε] > [α] or, in the constrained version, [ε] > [α] | [α] = 0.

Complex indicators raise several fundamental issues. One is the *basket* question: how many and which simple indicators to include in the complex indicator set or basket. Another is the manner in which the simple indicators are combined or weighted. These questions apply not only to the experimenter but also to the uninstructed subject interrogating his or her own consciousness. Thus it would be a mistake to view these questions as exclusively "problems" of methodology or theory for the experimenter; to the extent that they are problems for the uninstructed subject in everyday life, they become substantive psychological issues on their own right (Erdelyi 1985).

A still more complex form of complex indicators, hence *hypercomplex* indicators (Erdelyi 1985), arises from the interaction of simple indicators. A simple indicator event, ε, such as the statement, "Brutus is an honorable man," can carry more (or different) meanings when considered against a particular background context, [ε], than in isolation. Thus ε | [ε] > ε. This obvious fact, ubiquitously exemplified by complex polysemic forms such as jokes, irony, sarcasm, and poetry, lies at the heart of psychoanalytic psychology (see Erdelyi 1985). The distinction between surface (ε) and deeper meanings (ε | [ε]) is what Freud referred to as the distinction between *manifest* and *latent* content. What parlays Freud's distinction into a fabulous story—whether true or false—is his claim that in addition to the commonplace *conscious* double-meanings (in jokes, sarcasm, etc.) a person may also emit double-messages without being aware of their latent contents. Thus when the individual is conscious only of the surface content ($\alpha = \varepsilon$) the dissociation paradigm with hypercomplex indicators is realized when $\varepsilon \mid [\varepsilon] > \varepsilon$. This perhaps is the most important variant of *subliminal perception,* though it has been blatantly ignored by laboratory psychology—if not by Madison Avenue. The type of "perception" involved here is the one intended by expressions such as "seeing the point" or "seeing the connection"; it is sight in the sense of insight. Experimental psychology has tended to bypass this type of evidence because of its penchant for identifying the *stimulus* with palpable physical events (controlled by tachistoscopes, filters, masks, etc.) rather than psychological manipulations (such as context selection). The classic *limen* of Herbart and Fechner is a threshold of *consciousness* (or subjective sensation), not a *sensory* threshold, as seems to be widely assumed. Stimuli above this threshold are apprehended consciously; those below it are not. Hence the stimuli of interest need not be restricted to sensory inputs but can include constructions of the mind, such as latent contents, which may or may not be apprehended consciously. In the defense mechanism of denial, which is the hypercomplex variant of the classic perceptual defense, the person may be fully conscious of the surface event, ε, and all the constituents of the context, $[\varepsilon]$, yet be completely unaware of their interaction, $\varepsilon \mid [\varepsilon]$. The unconscious here is both invisible and complex. As in statistics, an exhaustive analysis of main effects may miss the interaction.

The Recovery Paradigm of the Unconscious

The recovery (of memory) paradigm is also a dissociation paradigm, one involving a temporal dissociation. In Hilgard's words, "Amnesia, as a temporary loss of memories that may be recovered, is the key to the understanding of dissociation" (Hilgard 1977, p. 62).

Formally, the recovery paradigm is realized when a second test of memory contains stimulus information not accessible in an earlier test, as in hypermnesia and reminiscence. It may be concluded from such a situation that the information was originally unconscious—dissociated from consciousness. Unlike the standard dissociation paradigm, involving two concurrent indicators, the recovery paradigm makes use of only one indicator, α, but the indicator is used more than once. Formally, if α_1 is an indicator of accessibility (such as recall) administered at time 1 and if α_2 is the same indicator probed on a second occasion, the recovery paradigm is realized when $\alpha_2 > \alpha_1$.

Despite some past controversies (see Erdelyi 1984; H. M. Erdelyi, unpublished observations, 1994), the phenomena of *reminiscence* (recovery of items in later trials that were not accessible on earlier ones) and *hypermnesia* (overall increase of memory from an earlier to a later test) have become undisputed (see Erdelyi 1984; H. M. Erdelyi, unpublished observations, 1994; Payne 1987; Roediger and Thorpe 1978). Such accessibility increments, as Ballard (1913) reluctantly acknowledged in his reference monograph, logically imply the existence of unconscious contents, for the recovered material has to come from somewhere. Hypermnesia and reminiscence effects are not only reliable but can be powerful. Erdelyi and Kleinbard (1978), for example, showed that recall level could increase between 50% and 100% over a week of protracted recall effort. It is therefore no longer implausible to believe that substantial memory recoveries are achieved in therapy, as psychodynamic clinicians have long claimed. Moreover, clinicians have observed recoveries of thought and action structures (schemas, scripts, complexes; see Horowitz 1991) that reach levels of complexity sufficient to invoke the designation of subpersonalities (e.g., Jung 1935/1968).

Memory effects—both amnesic and hypermnesic—have begun to emerge as a critical issue in the subception area. Put another way, the factor of *time* is beginning to be seen as critical. Thus Holender (1986) dismissed evidence for subliminal perception based on the dichotic listening design on the ground that awareness might have been present for the rejected stimulus at the time of the dichotic listening but forgotten by the time it was probed. Unfortunately, this argument poses a problem for all evidence based on the dissociation paradigm because some time must elapse in any perceptual report. The distinction between perception and memory, though often convenient, can also be misleading and is ultimately one of the pretheoretic notions that we have not yet superseded three decades into the information-processing approach to psychology (see Erdelyi 1974).

Forgetting, however, is not the only problem, because, to the extent that hypermnesia applies to subliminal stimuli, chance-level perception (absolute subliminality) at time 1 may become above-chance (supraliminal) perception at time 2. I (Erdelyi 1986) explicitly raised the possibility of a flip-flop effect in the KWZ phenomenon over time, wherein the chance-level direct measure would, over time, become above chance and the initially above-chance indirect measure would decline to chance. Merikle and Reingold (1991) tested this possibility and found just such an effect in two separate studies. Specifically, when they subdivided their overall recognition test into first, second, and third parts—block 1, block 2, and block 3—they found that what was chance-level recognition memory in the first two-thirds of the overall recognition test (blocks 1 and 2) became significantly above-chance recognition memory in block 3; the opposite was observed for an indirect measure of memory (subjective *contrast*), which went from above chance in block 1 to chance level by block 3. Thus even methodologically exacting demonstrations of *absolute subliminality* (e.g., where the accessibility measure, d', yields $d' = 0$) may apply only in certain (arbitrarily chosen) temporal windows. The recovery (temporal dissociation) paradigm impinges on the (concurrent) dissociation paradigm. Perhaps the distinction between conscious and unconscious, which like the perception versus memory distinction may be serviceable in a loose, pretheoretic sense, breaks down in formal analysis. What we may ultimately be left with are the basic paradigms, which may or may not map onto the fuzzy notion of conscious and unconscious.

The *unconscious* of the dissociation paradigm, for example, is really derived from the dissociation of two or more indicators *over a particular temporal window* (see Figure 1–1).

Different indicators—$\alpha(t)$, $\epsilon(t)$—may have different rise and fall characteristics over time. The arbitrary selection of a particular temporal window (e.g., Δt_1) can yield an unconscious effect—area under $\alpha(t) = 0$, under $\epsilon(t) > 0$—which disappears in a different temporal window (e.g., Δt_3; see Ionescu and Erdelyi 1992). Again, this is not just an experimental problem. It is a fundamental problem area in psychology. The subject's choice of indicators, baskets, combinations, temporal windows all fall under the aegis of psychodynamics. The *unconscious* is a pretheoretic term. The undergirding paradigms are the reality, and what experimentalists and clinicians observe only more or less captures the multidimensional events at play.

SUMMARY AND CONCLUSIONS

Dissociationism has had a long history in philosophy and psychology. It has been associated in dynamic psychology with polypsychism, the view that the unity of the self is an illusion and that the self actually constitutes a multiplicity of subselves. *Dissociation* is observed when the subselves lose cohesion and act in an independent or contradictory fashion. Both polypsychism (under labels such as *modularity)* and dissociationism are basic to contemporary psychology and neuroscience.

A general systems theory framework, which is adopted in this chapter, suggests that all complex systems—biological, psychological, and sociological—of necessity are polypsychist in the sense of subsuming subsystems that may become relatively dissociated. Thus discrepancies in the operation of subsystems are the phenomena that define dissociations within the superordinate system. Such dissociations underlie and ultimately define a va-

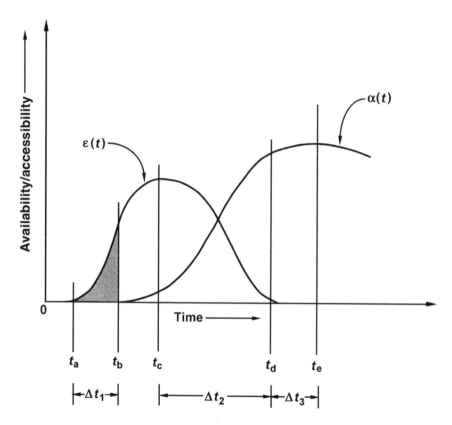

Figure 1–1. Rise and fall over time of two hypothetical measures, $\alpha(t)$ and $\varepsilon(t)$, of accessibility/availability. Dissociation between indicators is defined by the difference in subtended area, within a chosen temporal window, Δt_1, of the two indicator functions. The Kunst-Wilson and Zajonc (KWZ) effect is shown in temporal window Δt_1, which was obtained by Merikle and Reingold (1991) in block 1 of their testing. The flip-flop of the KWZ effect is illustrated by temporal window Δt_3 (block 3 of Merikle and Reingold).
Source. Adapted with permission from Ionescu MD, Erdelyi MH: "The Direct Recovery of Subliminal Stimuli," in *Perception Without Awareness.* Edited by Bornstein RF, Pittman TS. New York, Guilford, 1992, p. 165.

riety of central concepts in psychology, including the *unconscious* and *defense (the dynamic unconscious)*.

The latter portion of the chapter attempts to show, in some technical detail, how the unconscious, in its myriad manifestations, is reducible to two types of dissociations: concurrent dissociations and temporal dissociations of the hypermnesic variety.

REFERENCES

Ballard PB: Oblivescence and reminiscence. British Journal of Psychology: Monograph Supplements 1:1–82, 1913

Binet A: On Double Consciousness: Experimental Psychological Studies. Chicago, IL, Open Court Publishing Company, 1889–1890

Bornstein RF, Pittman TS (eds): Perception Without Awareness. New York, Guilford, 1992

Bowers KS: On being unconsciously influenced and informed, in The Unconscious Reconsidered. Edited by Bowers KS, Meichenbaum D. New York, Wiley, 1984, pp 227–272

Breuer J, Freud S: Studies on hysteria (1895), in The Standard Edition of the Complete Psychological Works of Sigmund Freud, Vol 2. Translated and edited and by Strachey J. London, Hogarth Press, 1955, pp 1–335

Dessoir M: Das Doppel-Ich (1890). Leipzig, Ernst Guenthers, 1986

Deutsch M: The Nerves of Government. New York, Free Press, 1966

Ebbinghaus H: Memory (1885). Translated by Ruger HA, Bussenius CE. New York, Dover, 1964

Ellenberger HF: The Discovery of the Unconscious. New York, Basic Books, 1970

Erdelyi MH: A new look at the New Look: perceptual defense and vigilance. Psychol Rev 81:1–25, 1974

Erdelyi MH: The recovery of unconscious (inaccessible) memories: laboratory studies of hypermnesia, in The Psychology of Learning and Motivation: Advances in Research and Theory, Vol 18. Edited by Bower G. New York, Academic Press, 1984, pp 95–127

Erdelyi MH: Psychoanalysis: Freud's Cognitive Psychology. New York, WH Freeman, 1985

Erdelyi MH: Experimental indeterminacies in the dissociation paradigm of subliminal perception. The Behavioral and Brain Sciences 9:30–31, 1986

Erdelyi MH: Repression, reconstruction, and defense: history and integration of the psychoanalytic and experimental frameworks, in Repression and Dissociation: Implications for Personality Theory, Psychopathology, and Health. Edited by Singer JL. Chicago, IL, Chicago University Press, 1990, pp 1–31

Erdelyi MH: Psychodynamics and the unconscious. Am Psychol 47:784–787, 1992

Erdelyi MH: Repression: the mechanism and the defense, in The Handbook of Mental Control. Edited by Wegner DM, Pennebaker JW. Englewood Cliffs, NJ, Simon & Schuster, 1993, pp 126–148

Erdelyi MH, Becker J: Hypermnesia for pictures: incremental memory for pictures but not words in multiple recall trials. Cognitive Psychology 6:159–171, 1974

Erdelyi MH, Kleinbard J: Has Ebbinghaus decayed with time? The growth of recall (hypermnesia) over days. Journal of Experimental Psychology: Human Learning and Memory 4:275–289, 1978

Eriksen CW: Unconscious processes, in Nebraska Symposium on Motivation. Edited by Jones MR. Lincoln, NE, University of Nebraska Press, 1958, pp 169–227

Fodor JA: The Modularity of Mind. Cambridge, MA, MIT Press, 1983

Freud S: The neuro-psychoses of defence (1894), in The Standard Edition of the Complete Psychological Works of Sigmund Freud, Vol 3. Translated and edited by Strachey J. London, Hogarth Press, 1962, pp 43–61

Freud S: The defense neuro-psychoses (1894), in Sigmund Freud: Early Psychoanalytic Writings. Translated by Rickman J. Edited by Rieff P. New York, Collier, 1963, pp 67–81

Freud S: The ego and the id (1923), in The Standard Edition of the Complete Psychological Works of Sigmund Freud, Vol 19. Translated and edited by Strachey J. London, Hogarth Press, 1961, pp 3–66

Freud S: New introductory lectures on psycho-analysis (1933), in The Standard Edition of the Complete Psychological Works of Sigmund Freud, Vol 20. Translated and edited by Strachey J. London, Hogarth Press, 1961, pp 3–182

Gazzaniga MS: The Social Brain. New York, Basic Books, 1985

Goldiamond I: Indicators of perception; I: subliminal perception, subception, unconscious perception: an analysis in terms of psychophysical methodology. Psychol Bull 55:373–411, 1958

Hilgard EB: Divided Consciousness: Multiple Controls in Human Thought and Action. New York, Wiley, 1977

Hobson JA: The Dreaming Brain. New York, Basic Books, 1988

Holender D: Semantic activation without conscious identification in dichotic listening, parafoveal vision, and visual masking: a survey and appraisal. The Behavioral and Brain Sciences 9:1–66, 1986

Horowitz MJ: Person Schemas and Maladaptive Interpersonal Patterns. Chicago, IL, University of Chicago Press, 1991

Ionescu MD, Erdelyi MH: The direct recovery of subliminal stimuli, in Perception Without Awareness. Edited by Bornstein RF, Pittman TS. New York, Guilford, 1992, pp 143–169

Janet P: L'Automatisme Psychologique. Paris, Felix Alcan, 1889

Jung CG: Analytical Psychology: Its Theory and Practice (1935). New York, Pantheon, 1968

Koestler A: The Ghost in the Machine. Chicago, IL, Henry Regnery, 1967

Kunst-Wilson WR, Zajonc RB: Affective discrimination of stimuli that cannot be recognized. Science 207:557–558, 1980

Lorenz K: On Aggression. Translated by Wilson MK. New York, Harcourt Brace Jovanovich, 1966

Lewandowsky S, Dunn JC, Krisner K (eds): Implicit Memory: Theoretical Issues. Hillsdale, NJ, Erlbaum, 1989

McGinnies E: Emotionality and perceptual defense. Psychol Rev 56:244–251, 1949

Macmillan NA: The psychophysics of subliminal perception. The Behavioral and Brain Sciences 9:38–39, 1986

Merikle PM, Cheesman J: Consciousness is a "subjective" state. The Behavioral and Brain Sciences 9:42–43, 1986

Merikle PM, Reingold EM: Comparing direct (explicit) and indirect (implicit) measures to study nonconscious memory. J Exp Psychol Learn Mem Cogn 17:224–233, 1991

Miller JG: Living Systems. New York, McGraw-Hill, 1978

Nemiah JC: The unconscious in psychopathology, in The Unconscious Reconsidered. Edited by Bowers KS, Meichenbaum D. New York, Wiley, 1984, pp 49–87

Parkin AJ: Memory and Amnesia: An Introduction. Oxford, Blackwell, 1987

Payne DG: Hypermnesia and reminiscence in recall: a historical and empirical review. Psychol Bull 101:5–27, 1987

Prince M: The Dissociation of Personality. New York, Longmans Green, 1906

Reingold EM, Merikle PM: Using direct and indirect measures to study perception and awareness. Perception and Psychophysics 44:563–575, 1988

Roediger HL, Thorpe LA: The role of recall time in producing hypermnesia. Memory and Cognition 6:296–305, 1978

Singer JL: Repression and Dissociation: Implications for Personality Theory, Psychopathology, and Health. Chicago, IL, University of Chicago Press, 1990

Uleman JS, Bargh JA (eds): Unintended Thought. New York, Guilford, 1989

Von Bertalanffy L: General Systems Theory: Foundations, Development, Application. New York, George Braziller, 1968

CHAPTER 2

Dissociated Control, Imagination, and the Phenomenology of Dissociation

Kenneth S. Bowers, Ph.D.

Generally speaking, there are three different kinds of experience associated with hypnotic phenomena (Woody et al. 1992): 1) the suggested effect per se (e.g., analgesia to painful stimuli, hallucinated sights and sounds), 2) the images and fantasies that typically accompany suggested effects (e.g., the counter-pain image, accompanying analgesia, that one's hand is like a block of wood, incapable of feeling pain), and 3) the experience of nonvolition that often accompanies suggested effects (e.g., the feeling that a hand is rising by itself).

Regarding the first of the above experiences, there historically has been considerable skepticism about the reality or genuineness of suggested effects. For example, one does not have to look very far to find venomous opposition to the effectiveness of hypnotic analgesia (K. S. Bowers 1983; Perry and Laurence 1983; Rosen 1946). Fortunately, skepticism has changed its face in the last decade or so. Spanos, for example, is on record as confirming the subjective reality of hypnotic analgesia (Spanos et al. 1979) and hypnotic amnesia (Spanos et al. 1980). In one recent article, Spanos (1987) asserted "the controversies . . . are not about whether hypnotic phenomena exist or are 'real.' Instead, they revolve around disagreement about the most useful ways of conceptualizing these phenomena and about which variables are thought to mediate hypnotic responding" (p. 778).

The controversy surrounding how best to conceptualize hypnotically suggested effects is, at least to some extent, a controversy about the evidential status of the other two kinds of subjective reports. Spanos gives prior importance to reports of various cognitions, such as imagery and goal-directed fantasies, which he regards as strategic enactments that help mediate hypnotic responses. According to this view, the nonvolitional experiences that hypnotized subjects report are consigned to evidential oblivion; they are simply regarded as misattributions of volitional acts to the hypnotic context and to concurrent fantasies and related cognitions (Spanos 1986).

A more traditional view of hypnosis asks us to take reports of nonvolition seriously as evidence for a dissociative process underlying hypnotic responses. Weitzenhoffer (1978) dubbed the nonvolitional quality of hypnotic responses the *classic suggestion effect* and has given it central importance in his conceptualization of hypnosis. But imagery and fantasy that ordinarily accompany hypnotically suggested effects are not dismissed by this more traditional view. Quite the contrary, the entire concept of imaginative involvement (J. R. Hilgard 1979), absorption (Tellegen and Atkinson 1974), or believed in imaginings (Sarbin and Coe 1972) has a long and honored place in this tradition.

A DILEMMA TO RESOLVE

There is, however, a seldom noticed dilemma that the traditional view must confront in its emphasis on both imaginative involvement and dissociation as critical to an understanding of hypnosis. The dilemma boils down to this: The emphasis on involved imagining implies that the *presence,* in conscious experience, of various ideas, images, and imaginings is critical to the production of hypnotic responding. On the other hand, the emphasis on dissociation has historically implied that the *absence,* from conscious experience, of various influential ideas, images, and imaginings is important to an understanding of hypnotic responding—and to an understanding of various dissociative disorders that are viewed as conceptually akin to hypnosis (Erdelyi 1985, 1990; Janet 1907/1965).

Investigators of a traditional persuasion have sometimes sensed this dilemma, but few have stated it as explicitly as Spiegel (1990), who commented that "it is not immediately obvious what the relation between absorption and dissociation is. While both are clearly associated with hypnotic experience, neither phenomenon seems able to account fully for the other" (p. 130). He then applies a connectionist model (Baars 1988) in an attempt to resolve this puzzlement. My attempt to resolve the matter has a very different emphasis, though at some level there are similarities in the two approaches.

One of the perplexities surrounding this issue is that although absorption and dissociation seem conceptually so distinct, it is extremely hard to separate them empirically. Thus measures of dissociation typically correlate much higher with measures of absorption (about .70) than either measure correlates with hypnotic ability (typically less than .30; e.g., Nadon et al. 1991). How can dissociation, implying a cognitive lacuna, be so empirically connected to absorption, which implies the presence—in spades—of conscious cognitive content?

Perhaps a closer examination of the concepts of dissociation and absorption will help to resolve the dilemma.

DISSOCIATION AS AMNESIA

In his 1977 book, *Divided Consciousness,* E. R. Hilgard proposed at least two possible dissociative mechanisms. One of them depends on an amnesia-like process in which specific sensations and/or mental content are temporarily hidden from consciousness. The second mechanism does not involve amnesia in any strict sense. Rather, it involves an alteration in the hierarchy of cognitive control generating thought and action. I will focus mostly on this second notion of dissociation.

First of all, however, I want to propose that—at least in the context of hypnosis—the amnestic basis for dissociation is not at all well established. To be sure, dissociation implies that certain mental events and/or processes are not consciously represented, but I am unconvinced that amnesia—at least as it is ordinarily understood—is the best way of understanding this lack of consciousness. Consider, for example, the possible role of amnesia in the hypnotic control of pain. In one of Hilgard's many experiments on hypnotic analgesia (E. R. Hilgard et al. 1975), some subjects who were hypnotically analgesic for a painful stimulus retrospectively recalled pain levels appropriate to the stimulus intensity. According to the authors, this finding implies subjects' amnesia for pain that was covertly experienced in parallel with analgesia for it. There are, however, some difficulties associated with this proposal.

First, in this and related experiments, amnesia was not explicitly suggested. But unsuggested, spontaneous amnesia in normal laboratory subjects is extremely rare (E. R. Hilgard and Cooper 1965), far more so than the analgesia it presumably explains. Accordingly, it is not at all clear how something rare can routinely account for a phenomenon that is relatively common. Second, Hilgard himself appreciates that whereas some sort of amnesia may be involved in hypnotic analgesia, "it is an amnesia for something that has not been in awareness previously, [so] it differs from usual posthypnotic amnesia" (E. R. Hilgard et al. 1975, p. 288). However, the nature of this difference is not further specified.

There is a third difficulty with an amnestic account of analgesia: According to Hilgard, generating amnesia for information that would ordinarily be conscious requires considerable cognitive effort that in turn impairs performance on a concomitant, consciously performed task (e.g., Stevenson 1976). However, recent research conducted in our laboratory strongly implies that hypnotically suggested analgesia does *not* detract from performance on such a task (Miller and Bowers 1993). This finding casts doubt on the assumption that hypnotic analgesia involves cognitive work to keep painful sensations out of awareness.

Although the above considerations do not completely disallow an amnestic basis for dissociation, they do establish the need for strong counterarguments to sustain it—at least in the context of hypnotic analgesia. Part of the problem is that we need a better way of thinking about how consciousness, memory, and amnesia are interrelated. For instance, it seems unlikely that all cases in which a person is not conscious of information or stimulation are best understood as being due to amnesia. Accordingly, it is reasonable to ask: What besides amnesia can reduce or eliminate consciousness of various mental content or processes? A related question might be: What kind of mental content or processes can be dissociated from consciousness, whether by amnesia or not? These are complex questions that I cannot fully address in this chapter but which certainly deserve a full and systematic account.

This chapter has a more limited goal, namely, to focus on the implications of nonvolitional experience as it is relevant to an understanding of dissociation. I argue that such an experience represents the absence, from consciousness, of the sense of agency and personal initiative that ordinarily informs everyday behavior, thereby qualifying as an example of dissociation. The question is how best to understand such nonvolitional experience.

DISSOCIATED CONTROL

Although Hilgard certainly proposes amnesia as a basis for dissociation, I think it is fair to say that the major thrust of his thinking is better captured by the notion of *dissociated control* (K. S. Bowers 1990, 1991, 1992a, 1992b). Human cognition is conceived as having a hierarchical nature, with lower subsystems of control ordinarily being responsive to the highest levels of control (i.e., to executive initiative and monitoring). These subsystems of control can be viewed as overlearned action/experience modules or schemas that do not require much attention in order to be activated. Thus dialing a familiar phone number can occur without much thought or attention. Indeed, a familiar phone number is occasionally dialed instead of the intended one (see Heckhausen and Beckmann 1990; Norman 1981; Reason 1979), an eventuality that was portrayed as a pivotal incident in Tom Wolfe's (1987) novel, *The Bonfire of the Vanities*. Near the beginning of the book the main character inadvertently calls his wife instead of his lover. His wife instantly realizes the nature of the mistake, and all hell breaks loose. Ordinarily, of course, subsystems of control are organized by higher levels of control into action sequences that are part of planned, purposeful behavior.

By my understanding of Hilgard's (1977) neodissociation model, subsystems of control can be activated by hypnotic suggestions more or less directly, without involving higher levels of control (see Miller et al. 1960). Because executive initiative and effort is ordinarily experienced as volitional, and because hypnotically suggested behavior tends to bypass such high-level executive control, hypnotic responses are typically experienced as nonvolitional. In effect, lower subsystems of control have been dissociated from high-level executive work, which is why I refer to this process as *dissociated control* (K. S. Bowers 1990, 1991, 1992a, 1992b).

Notice that for the hypnotized subject, the suggestive communication and the behavioral response to it remain conscious; absent from consciousness is the willful connection that ordinarily links behavior to its antecedents and anticipated outcomes. However, the fact that the experience of volition is not consciously represented does not imply amnesia for it. Clearly, if executive initiative is not the impetus to action in the first place, it is simply not subject to subsequent forgetting or recall. In sum, the experience of nonvolition that ordinarily accompanies a hypnotic response exemplifies one nonamnestic basis of dissociation.

THE LIMITATIONS OF IMAGINATIVE INVOLVEMENT/ABSORPTION

Now let us turn to the notion of imaginative involvement. The evidence for the mediating impact of imaginative involvement on hypnotic responsiveness rests for the most part on two kinds of evidence: 1) retrospective reports by hypnotized subjects of fantasies or imaginings that seem strategically produced to engender suggested effects, for example, a report by a hypnotically analgesic subject that his or her hand was, per suggestion, made of wood (e.g., E. R. Hilgard and J. R. Hilgard 1975; J. R. Hilgard and LeBaron 1984; Spanos et al. 1979); and 2) the correlation of hypnotic ability with subjects' reports of unusual and unrealistic experiences in everyday life (e.g., Shor 1979; Tellegen and Atkinson 1974).

Is Imagination a Mediator of Hypnotic Responding?

With regard to the first type of evidence, various investigations indicate that instructed increases in goal-directed fantasy (Spanos 1971) do *not* enhance hypnotic responsiveness (e.g., Buckner and Coe 1977; Lynn et al. 1983; Lynn et al. 1987; Spanos and McPeake 1974). Indeed, subjects can respond behaviorally to suggestions that are concurrently *contradicted* by various suggested thoughts and imaginings (Bartis and Zamansky 1990; Zamansky 1977; Zamansky and Clark 1986). In addition, two recent investigations from our laboratory cast additional doubt on the notion that imagery and imagination mediate hypnotic responding.

Miller and Bowers (1986) found that regardless of hypnotizability, very few hypnotized subjects reported the strategic use of counter-pain imagery. Nevertheless, *high-hypnotizable* subjects were far more successful in reducing pain than their *low-hypnotizable* counterparts. In contrast, imagery and other cognitive strategies did seem to mediate the reduced pain of both high- and low-hypnotizable subjects who were not hypnotized but who were instead trained to use stress inoculation techniques (e.g., Turk et al. 1983) to cope with pain. In other words, various cognitive strategies, in-

26

cluding counter-pain imagery, do reduce pain. However, such strategies do not seem to be the *modus operandi* of hypnotic analgesia.

In a later publication, Miller and Bowers (1993) reported more direct evidence that strategies of pain control (including counter-pain imagery) were less characteristic of hypnotic analgesia than they were for stress inoculation. As subjects attempted to reduce cold pressor pain in one of these two ways, they simultaneously performed a cognitively demanding task. Stress-inoculation subjects showed about a 30% decrease in the performance on this secondary task from a pretreatment level of performance (in which subjects' forearms were submitted to cold pressor), indicating that the pain reductions thus achieved had associated cognitive costs. Hypnotic-analgesia subjects were as successful in reducing pain as their stress-inoculation counterparts but with no loss in their ability to perform the secondary task. If hypnotic analgesia had involved cognitive work (such as deliberately invoking counter-pain imagery), their performance on the secondary task should have been impaired, just as it was for subjects in the stress inoculation condition. This was not the case. Evidently, hypnotic analgesia is not simply a matter of "motivated subjects actively coping with . . . noxious stimulation" (Spanos 1986, p. 458).

In her dissertation, Debra Hughes (1988) followed up some earlier work by John Lacey (1967), which demonstrated that changes in heart rate indexed cognitive work. Of particular interest for present purposes, Lacey found that when attention was internally focused, heart rate increased. Effortfully generating internal imagery should thus generate increases in heart rate, which could thus serve as an independent index of such cognitive work.

Hughes found that even though 30 high-hypnotizable subjects reported far more vivid neutral imagery than their 30 low-hypnotizable counterparts, there was no corresponding difference in the amount of heart rate increase from a preimagery baseline. Therefore, at least according to this cardiac criterion of cognitive effort, high-hypnotizable subjects worked no harder than low-hypnotizable subjects to produce much more vivid imagery.

Further analyses revealed that low-hypnotizable subjects who engaged in hypnotically suggested imagery showed the expected positive relationship (Pearson's *r* of approximately .50) between ratings of cognitive effort and heart rate increase—a relationship that held for both neutral and fear imagery. Thus for low-hypnotizable subjects, the more rated effort involved in generating imagery, the more heart rate increased from a nonimagery baseline. This outcome is exactly what a social psychological position would predict. However, the situation was quite otherwise for the high-hyp-notizable subjects: In the neutral imagery condition they showed no rela-tionship at all between the heart rate index and ratings of the cognitive effort involved in producing imagery; when fear imagery was suggested, the correlation between these two variables was −.52, indicating that the *less* effort expended to produce the imagery, the *more* heart rate increased. Internal analysis of the data strongly implied that for high-hypnotizable subjects the heart rate increases associated with the production of fear im-agery indexed emotional arousal rather than the cognitive effort involved in producing the imagery (a more extended summary of Hughes's findings can be found in K. S. Bowers 1991). Upon reflection, it is not surprising that when hypnotically suggested fear imagery is experienced as *not* being under conscious executive control, the outcome is apt to be particularly frightening.

To summarize the above findings: In contrast to low-hypnotizable sub-jects, suggested imagery in high-hypnotizable subjects does not seem to be strategically or effortfully enacted; instead, the imagery seems to be directly activated by the suggestions and has all the familiar character of the *classic suggestion effect* (Weitzenhoffer 1978)—namely, a peremptory, nonvolitio-nal quality. When fear imagery is suggested, its resulting "out-of-control" quality can be especially frightening. However, not only imagery but other hypnotic responses such as analgesia can be directly activated. Accordingly, if both counter-pain images and reduced pain are each directly activated by hypnotic suggestion, the implication is that counter-pain images simply co-occur with the analgesia rather than mediate it (see Buckner and Coe 1977). We shall return to this theme shortly.

The above evidence calls into question the importance of strategically produced fantasy or imaginative involvement as mediators of hypnotically suggested effects—especially in high-hypnotizable subjects. This is not to deny that such imagery often accompanies suggested effects.

Correlations of Hypnotic Ability and Absorption

The second type of evidence that seems to support an intimate association of imagery and hypnotic responsiveness is the modest but consistent cor-relations of hypnotic ability and unusual experiences in everyday life. There have been many ways of tapping unusual real-life experiences (e.g., Glisky et al. 1991; J. R. Hilgard 1979; Nadon et al. 1987; Shor 1979), but the Telle-gen Absorption Scale (TAS; Tellegen and Atkinson 1974) is the most common means of doing so. Balthazard and Woody (1992) recently presented data indicating that the TAS, though correlating very modestly with the entire range of hypnotic ability (e.g., De Groh 1989; Nadon et al. 1991), accounts for most of the variance in high-end hypnotizability (see also K. S. Bowers 1971; Isaacs 1982; Shor et al. 1962; Woody et al. 1992). Notice that on strictly statistical grounds, *if* hypnotizability were unidimensional, restricting its range should decrease, not increase, the magnitude of correlation between it and the TAS. The fact that the correlation between these two variables is considerably higher among high-hypnotizable subjects than it is across the entire range of hypnotic ability is powerful evidence that hypnotizability is not unidimensional (see Monteiro et al. 1980). In any case, how can we reconcile evidence for the correlation of absorption and hypnotic ability on the one hand with findings that imaginative involvement seems very limited as a mediator of hypnotic responsiveness on the other?

DISSOCIATED CONTROL VERSUS IMAGINATIVE INVOLVEMENT AS THE BASIS FOR HYPNOTIC RESPONDING

Assume for a moment that hypnotized individuals do in fact achieve suggested analgesia by dissociated control. According to a neodissociative account of hypnosis, their reductions in pain are more or less directly activated by hypnotic suggestions. However, suggestions for analgesia typically include images designed to help subjects reduce pain (e.g., a suggestion that "your arm is like wood"). Therefore, when subjects subsequently mention the occurrence of such images, it is easy to assume that they helped mediate analgesia. However, insofar as pain reduction was actually achieved by dissociated control, these images and imaginings have the status of concomitants rather than mediators of suggested analgesia. Because people who are more hypnotically responsive to suggestions for analgesia are also apt to be more responsive to suggestions for imagery, hypnotic analgesia and the extent or vividness of imagery should be correlated.

Let me take this relationship one step further. In a manner that may at first seem paradoxical, the less fantasy actually mediates pain reduction, the more in evidence it may be, and for the following reason: *The more that pain is effectively reduced by dissociated control, the more high-level cognitive resources remain available for fantasy and involved imagining.* To be sure, the strategic use of imagery, imagination, and related techniques is effective in reducing pain (Marino et al. 1989; Turk et al. 1983). However, conscious mobilization of such counter-pain strategies may well be vulnerable to distractions and to competing demands on high-level cognitive resources (Farthing et al. 1984; Miller and Bowers 1993). Thus severe pain could well distract attention from the strategic efforts (e.g., imagery, fantasies) deployed to reduce it (McCaul and Malott 1984).

If the above account has some validity, the most hypnotically analgesic subjects will ordinarily report the most imaginative involvement. However, this correlation would imply that imaginative involvement reflects the dissociated control of pain, *not* that such involvement mediates analgesia. Moreover, the propensity to engage in dissociated control may well be most developed in subjects of high hypnotic ability (K. S. Bowers 1990). Accordingly, the higher one's hypnotizability, the more cognitive resources would be available to become imaginatively involved while engaging in dissociated control of thought and action. This state of affairs would account for the modest but consistent correlation between hypnotic ability and individuals' scores on various experience inventories, such as the TAS.

Let us further assume that suggestion-induced dissociated control is more or less confined to high-hypnotizable subjects but that the propensity for such dissociated control varies directly with the degree of hypnotizability within this restricted range. Therefore, insofar as the TAS and related scales tap an imaginative factor that serves specifically as a marker of dissociation rather than as a mediator of suggested effects, the correlation between TAS-type scales and hypnotic ability should be higher within high-hypnotizable subjects than for the entire range of hypnotic ability. As mentioned earlier, there is in fact evidence of a potentiated relationship of hypnotizability and the TAS in subjects of relatively high hypnotic ability.

IMAGELESS ANALGESIA: A PRELIMINARY EXAMPLE

Suppose dissociated control and not imaginative involvement serves as the underlying mechanism of pain reduction. If that were so, high-hypnotizable subjects who are given suggestions to reduce pain without counter-pain imagery should be as analgesic as they would be to conventional (i.e., image-laden) hypnotic suggestions for hypnotic analgesia. That is, insofar as counter-pain images and fantasies are simply concomitants rather than mediators of hypnotic analgesia, eliminating or minimizing them via suggestion should not impair the degree of hypnotic analgesia.

Robin Hargadon, a graduate student in our laboratory, recently conducted a preliminary investigation with 14 high-hypnotizable subjects to see whether imageless analgesia does in fact occur (Hargadon and Bowers 1991). It is not irrelevant to mention here that several informed colleagues were quite skeptical about whether we would even find such a phenomenon—so ingrained is the assumption that relevant imagery mediates suggested effects. Nevertheless, 7 of the 14 subjects showed 44% more overall reduction of pain with imageless than with standard analgesia suggestions. Three of these 7 subjects later testified at some length about how much easier it was simply to turn off the pain rather than trying to minimize it via appropriate, counter-pain imagery. Here are some examples of how imagery was regarded by these subjects.

In describing her reaction to imageless analgesia, one subject said,

> I didn't feel anything in the hand—like nothing was there—inanimate. I didn't picture anything, nothing popped in to my head. I didn't picture a glove. I knew it was my hand, but I couldn't feel anything. I didn't imagine it was stone or wood. I put my hand in the [finger pressure device] and didn't feel anything for a while. Really neat. I wasn't even sure the bar was on my finger.

When asked how imageless analgesia compared with standard analgesia that included suggestions for contra-pain imagery, this same subject said,

> Not imagining anything is easier than trying to imagine there is something there. It worked better. Much better, just blocking. Much easier than imagining. The difference was astonishing . . . . It was just much easier not to think of anything at all because [I was] then not worried about the image fading in and out . . . . Just much easier and more enjoyable.

Another subject said, comparing imageless with standard analgesia,

> It seemed the less I did anything, like concentrate, the easier it was—more effective . . . . The second time, I was concentrating on do this, do that. It works, but not as effectively as the time when I was letting everything pass by. So I think the best thing is to let everything pass by you and not even think about anything.

The third subject, also comparing imageless with standard analgesia, said,

> [During the trial] I felt I had to really concentrate the whole time—I was imagining heat coming down to my hand and stopping the pain. Then when it got down to my hand I was imagining that I had a glove on. But I had to do that the whole time. I couldn't just relax like [the first time when] I didn't have to do anything. This time I really had to concentrate . . . . The first time—it was weird—I was just gone—I didn't feel anything. It was incredible. I was really gone. I didn't feel anything . . . . The second time, I really had to work at it. It worked as well, but I really had to work at it.

In sum, Hargadon's preliminary study indicated that in high-hypnotizable subjects imageless analgesia is superior to conventional (image-laden) suggestions for hypnotic analgesia about 50% of the time. In a major follow-up study using 66 carefully selected high-hypnotizable subjects, Hargadon and Bowers (1992) recently reported that imageless analgesia reduces pain to the same extent as conventional (image-laden) suggestions for analgesia. This finding casts further doubt on involved imagining as the mechanism of hypnotic responding; rather, it seems to be a marker of dissociated control.

IMPLICATIONS OF THE DISTINCTION BETWEEN DISSOCIATED CONTROL AND COGNITIVE STRATEGIES

What are some implications of the distinction between hypnotic responsiveness achieved by dissociated control on the one hand and by cognitive strategies (including deliberate use of counter-pain imagery) on the other? In the context of the clinical control of pain by hypnotic analgesia, my hunch is that both dissociated control and image-mediated reductions will be effective in acute, short-term pain—such as might be confronted at a dental office (see also Hilgard and LeBaron 1984). However, conscious mobilization of counter-pain imagery is very fatiguing if prolonged (McCaul and Mallot 1984). Moreover, as mentioned earlier, executive efforts to maintain strategic reductions in pain are probably subject to various distractions and challenges to the limited capacity characterizing conscious attention and control (Farthing et al. 1984; Shiffrin and Schneider 1977). Among these distractions, of course, is the very pain that strategically mobilized fantasy is designed to reduce.

On the other hand, perhaps such counter-pain imagery does not require ongoing effort to maintain it; instead, such imagery may simply sustain its own momentum—like a boulder rolling down a hill (see P. Bowers 1978; K. S. 1991). Even if that were true, however, ongoing involvement in fantasy is not a coping option that is completely compatible with reacting effectively to the challenges of everyday life. To illustrate, in their article on fantasy proneness, Wilson and Barber (1983) indicate that people who are capable of becoming profoundly absorbed in fantasy often use their talent as a temporary escape from reality. Indeed, the authors recount one woman who as a child placed herself in extreme jeopardy by walking on a busy highway that she fantasized was a country meadow.

Dissociated control of pain, on the other hand, implies that a subsystem of pain control can be more or less directly activated by suggestion, thereby forgoing the need for fantasy-mediated pain reduction. As the quotations of the subjects in Hargadon's previously mentioned study indicate, there seems to be an effortless quality to the reductions in pain thus achieved. It remains to be seen whether disconnecting from the pain in this fashion can sustain itself for long periods, but there are anecdotal reports in the literature to this effect. My hunch is that high-hypnotizable subjects capable of dissociated control can effectively minimize long-term chronic pain and do so in a way that does not impair effective adaptation to the vagaries of everyday life. However, I wish to stress the speculative nature of this hunch because, as far as I know, there is no adequately controlled investigation of the effect of hypnotic analgesia on protracted pain.

Another implication of dissociated control is that direct activation of low-level control limits the flexibility of the resulting behavior. One of the main advantages of high-level executive initiative and control is that it enables flexible adaptation to changing circumstances. That is, consciousness activates and integrates various subsystems of control in light of complex and changing circumstances, thereby increasing the chance that the person will behave flexibly and adaptively. However, when a relatively low level of control is directly activated, the resulting behavior has a more ballistic character—that is, its "flight path" is relatively unresponsive to considerations of context and appropriateness (see K. S. Bowers 1992a). Let me illustrate what I mean by returning briefly to *The Bonfire of the Vanities*. In the novel, the protagonist made rather elaborate attempts to elude his wife's detection, but this very preoccupation with his wife seems—at a critical moment—to have activated the dialing of her telephone number rather than that of his mistress. The unresponsiveness of this controlled sequence of behavior to high-level plans and intentions was his undoing and the making of a novel.

As we have seen, high-hypnotizable individuals seem particularly prone to have low levels of control directly activated by hypnotic suggestion. The presumed advantage to them is that the relatively ballistic outcome of an activated subsystem can engender analgesia (say) that high levels of initiative, effort, and control could also achieve, but not without being vulnerable to distraction and/or fatigue. We seem to have a potential trade-off here between flexibility and specificity. The higher and more flexible the control invoked, the more fatigue and distraction are apt to be competing influences and the less fixed outcomes are likely. However, when fixed outcomes are required, the more advantageous direct activation of lower control systems is apt to be. Which of these alternatives is most appropriate will, of course, depend on circumstances.

SUMMARY

To summarize my position briefly: Dissociated control of experience and action occurs when relatively low-level subsystems of control are more or less directly activated by hypnotic suggestion (see Miller et al. 1960). Such direct activation requires relatively little cognitive capacity. In contrast, a great deal of the lore in hypnosis, if not a great deal of evidence, emphasizes the importance of imaginative involvement as a strategic mediator of hypnotic responding. However, absorption and imaginative involvement may instead serve as a marker of dissociated control rather than as the mechanism of hypnotic responding. By this understanding, imagery and goal-directed fantasies are themselves more or less directly activated by hypnotic suggestion and are therefore concomitants of other hypnotically suggested effects (such as analgesia) rather than mediators of them. If this general view is correct, it will have important implications for reappraising past research that explores the relationship between hypnotic ability on one hand and imagery, absorption, and fantasy-proneness on the other.

REFERENCES

Baars BJ: A Cognitive Theory of Consciousness. Cambridge, Cambridge University Press, 1988

Balthazard CG, Woody EZ: The spectral analysis of hypnotic performance with respect to "absorption." Int J Clin Exp Hypn 40:21–43, 1992

Bartis SP, Zamansky HS: Cognitive strategies in hypnosis toward resolving the hypnotic conflict. Int J Clin Exp Hypn 38:168–182, 1990

Bowers KS: Sex and susceptibility as moderator variables in the relationship of creativity and hypnotic susceptibility. J Abnorm Psychol 78:93–100, 1971

Bowers KS: Hypnosis for the Seriously Curious. New York, Norton, 1983

Bowers KS: Unconscious influences and hypnosis, in Repression and Dissociation: Implications for Personality Theory, Psychopathology, and Health. Edited by Singer JL. Chicago, IL, University of Chicago Press, 1990, pp 143–178

Bowers KS: Dissociation in hypnosis and multiple personality disorder. Int J Clin Exp Hypn 39:155–176, 1991

Bowers KS: Dissociated control and the limits of hypnotic responsiveness. Consciousness and Cognition 1:32–39, 1992a

Bowers KS: Imagination and dissociative control in hypnotic responding. Int J Clin Exp Hypn 40:253–275, 1992b

Bowers P: Hypnotizability, creativity, and the role of effortless experiencing. Int J Clin Exp Hypn 26:184–202, 1978

Buckner LG, Coe WC: Imaginative skill, wording of suggestions, and hypnotic susceptibility. Int J Clin Exp Hypn 25:27–35, 1977

De Groh M: Correlates of hypnotic ability, in Hypnosis: The Cognitive-Behavioral Perspective. Edited by Spanos NP, Chaves JF. Buffalo, NY, Prometheus, 1989, pp 32–63

Erdelyi M: Psychoanalysis: Freud's Cognitive Psychology. New York, WH Freeman, 1985

Erdelyi MH: Repression, reconstruction, and defense: history and integration of the psychoanalytic and experimental frameworks, in Repression and Dissociation: Implications for Personality Theory, Psychopathology, and Health. Edited by Singer JL. Chicago, IL, University of Chicago Press, 1990, pp 1–32

Farthing GW, Venturino M, Brown SW: Suggestion and distraction in the control of pain: test of two hypotheses. J Abnorm Psychol 93:266–276, 1984

Glisky ML, Tataryn DJ, Tobias BA, et al: Absorption, openness to experience, and hypnotizability. J Pers Soc Psychol 60:263–272, 1991

Hargadon RM, Bowers KS: Hypnosis, instructional set, and stress inoculation: pain reduction and nonvolition. Paper presented at the annual meeting of the Society for Clinical and Experimental Hypnosis, New Orleans, LA, October 11, 1991

Hargadon RM, Bowers KS: High hypnotizables and hypnotic analgesia: an examination of underlying mechanisms. Paper presented at annual meeting of the Society for Clinical and Experimental Hypnosis, Washington, DC, October 23, 1992

Heckhausen H, Beckmann J: Intentional action and action slips. Psychol Rev 97:36–48, 1990

Hilgard ER: Divided Consciousness: Multiple Controls in Human Thought and Action. New York, Wiley, 1977

Hilgard ER, Cooper LM: Spontaneous and suggested post-hypnotic amnesia. Int J Clin Exp Hypn 13:261–273, 1965

Hilgard ER, Hilgard JR: Hypnosis in the Relief of Pain. Los Altos, CA, William Kaufmann, 1975

Hilgard ER, Morgan AH, Macdonald H: Pain and dissociation in the cold pressor test: a study of hypnotic analgesia with "hidden reports" through automatic key pressing and automatic talking. J Abnorm Psychol 84:280–289, 1975

Hilgard JR: Personality and Hypnosis: A Study of Imaginative Involvement, 2nd Edition. Chicago, IL, University of Chicago Press, 1979

Hilgard JR, LeBaron S: Hypnotherapy of Pain in Children With Cancer. Los Altos, CA, William Kaufmann, 1984

Hughes D: Factors related to heart rate change for high and low hypnotizables during imagery. Unpublished doctoral dissertation, University of Waterloo, Waterloo, Ontario, 1988

Isaacs P: Hypnotic responsiveness and dimensions of imagery and thinking style. Unpublished doctoral dissertation, University of Waterloo, Waterloo, Ontario, 1982

Janet P: Major Symptoms of Hysteria (1907). New York, Hafner, 1965

Lacey J: Somatic response patterning and stress: some revisions of activation theory, in Psychological Stress. Edited by Appley MH, Trumbell R. New York, Appleton-Century-Crofts, 1967, pp 14–37

Lynn SJ, Nash MR, Rhue JW, et al: Hypnosis and the experience of nonvolition. Int J Clin Exp Hypn 31:293–308, 1983

Lynn SJ, Snodgrass M, Rhue JW, et al: Goal-directed fantasy, hypnotic susceptibility, and expectancies. J Pers Soc Psychol 53:933–938, 1987

Marino J, Gwynn MI, Spanos NP: Cognitive mediators in the reduction of pain: the role of expectancy, strategy use, and self-presentation. J Abnorm Psychol 98:256–262, 1989

McCaul KD, Mallot JM: Distraction and coping with pain. Psychol Bull 95:516–533, 1984

Miller ME, Bowers KS: Hypnotic analgesia and stress inoculation in the reduction of pain. J Abnorm Psychol 95:6–14, 1986

Miller ME, Bowers KS: Hypnotic analgesia: dissociated experience or dissociated control? J Abnorm Psychol 102:29–38, 1993

Miller GA, Galanter E, Pribram KH: Plans and the Structure of Behavior. New York, Holt, 1960

Monteiro KP, Macdonald H, Hilgard ER: Imagery, absorption, and hypnosis: a factorial study. Journal of Mental Imagery 4:63–81, 1980

Nadon R, Laurence J, Perry C: Multiple predictors of hypnotic susceptibility. J Pers Soc Psychol 53:948–960, 1987

Nadon R, Hoyt IP, Register PA, et al: Absorption and hypnotizability: context effects reexamined. J Pers Soc Psychol 60:144–153, 1991

Norman D: Categorization of action slips. Psychol Rev 88:1–15, 1981

Perry C, Laurence J-R: Hypnosis, surgery, and mind-body interaction: an historical evaluation. Canadian Journal of Behavioral Science 15:351–372, 1983

Reason J: Actions not as planned: the price of automatization, in Aspects of Consciousness, Vol 1. Edited by Underwood G, Steven R. New York, Academic Press, 1979, pp 67–89

Rosen G: Mesmerism and surgery: a strange chapter in the history of anesthesia. Journal of the History of Medicine 1:527–550, 1946

Sarbin TL, Coe WC: Hypnosis: A Social Psychological Analysis of Influence Communication. New York, Holt, Rinehart, and Winston, 1972

Shiffrin RM, Schneider W: Controlled and automatic human information processing; II: perceptual learning, automatic attending, and a general theory. Psychol Rev 84:127–190, 1977

Shor RE: A phenomenological method for the measurement of variables important to an understanding of the nature of hypnosis, in Hypnosis: Developments in Research and New Perspectives, 2nd Edition. Edited by Fromm E, Shor RE. New York, Aldine, 1979, pp 105–135

Shor RE, Orne MT, O'Connell DN: Validation and cross-validation of a scale of self-reported personal experiences which predicts hypnotizability. J Psychol 53:55–75, 1962

Spanos NP: Goal-directed fantasy and the performance of hypnotic test suggestions. Psychiatry 34:86–96, 1971

Spanos NP: Hypnotic behavior: a social-psychological interpretation of amnesia, analgesia, and "trance logic." Behavioral and Brain Sciences 9:449–467, 1986

Spanos NP: Hypnotic behavior: special process accounts are still not required. Behavioral and Brain Sciences 10:776–781, 1987

Spanos NP, McPeake JD: Involvement in suggestion-related imaginings, experienced involuntariness, and credibility assigned to imaginings in hypnotic subjects. J Abnorm Psychol 83:687–690, 1974

Spanos NP, Radtke-Bodorik HL, Ferguson JD, et al: The effects of hypnotic susceptibility, suggestions for analgesia, and the utilization of cognitive strategies on the reduction of pain. J Abnorm Psychol 88:282–292, 1979

Spanos NP, Radtke-Bodorik L, Stam H: Disorganized recall during suggested amnesia: fact not artifact. J Abnorm Psychol 89:1–19, 1980

Spiegel D: Hypnosis, dissociation, and trauma: hidden and overt observers, in Repression and Dissociation: Implications for Personality Theory, Psychopathology, and Health. Edited by Singer JL. Chicago, IL, University of Chicago Press, 1990, pp 121–142

Stevenson JH: The effect of posthypnotic dissociation on the performance of interfering tasks. J Abnorm Psychol 85:398–407, 1976

Tellegen A, Atkinson G: Openness to absorbing and self-altering experiences ("absorption"), a trait related to hypnotic susceptibility. J Abnorm Psychol 83:268–277, 1974

Turk D, Meichenbaum DH, Genest M: Pain and Behavioral Medicine: A Cognitive-Behavioral Perspective. New York, Guilford, 1983

Weitzenhoffer AM: Hypnotism and altered states of consciousness, in Expanding Dimensions of Consciousness. Edited by Sugarman AA, Tarter RE. New York, Springer, 1978, pp 183–225

Wilson SC, Barber TX: The fantasy-prone personality: implications for understanding imagery, hypnosis, and parapsychological phenomena, in Imagery: Current Theory, Research, and Application. Edited by Sheikh AA. New York, Wiley, 1983, pp 340–390

Wolfe T: The Bonfire of the Vanities. New York, Farrar, Strauss & Giroux, 1987

Woody EZ, Bowers KS, Oakman JM: A conceptual analysis of hypnotic responsiveness: experience, individual differences and context, in Contemporary Perspectives in Hypnosis Research. Edited by Fromm E, Nash M. New York, Guilford, 1992, pp 3–33

Zamansky HS: Suggestion and countersuggestion. J Abnorm Psychol 86:346–351, 1977

Zamansky HS, Clark LE: Cognitive competition and hypnotic behavior: whither absorption. Int J Clin Exp Hypn 34:205–214, 1986

Section II

Measuring Dissociation

Studying the Interaction Between Physical and Psychological States With the Dissociative Experiences Scale

Eve B. Carlson, Ph.D.

S ince its publication in 1986, the Dissociative Experiences Scale (DES; Bernstein and Putnam 1986) has been used to study dissociation in a wide variety of contexts. This chapter focuses on areas of research that relate to the interaction between physical and psychological states. The research falls into four broad categories: 1) how dissociation is best defined and measured, 2) the relationship between dissociation and hypnotizability, 3) the relationship between dissociation and various physical states and conditions, and 4) the use of the DES in translation.

DEFINING AND MEASURING DISSOCIATION

In empirical research, the definitions and measurement of psychological phenomena are intricately and inextricably entwined. Whenever a psychological phenomenon is measured, some definition of the phenomenon is necessarily intrinsic to the measure. In this way, our understanding of dissociation is, in part, shaped by the scales we use to measure it. The definition of *dissociation* incorporated into the DES was intentionally broad. The authors attempted to include as wide a range of items as possible in the DES and tried to avoid including items that also measured some other distinct construct (such as modulation of affect). Consequently, the authors included many different kinds of experiences that had been previously associated with dissociation. There are items inquiring about amnestic experiences, gaps in awareness, depersonalization, derealization, absorption, and imaginative involvement. If the scale is an accurate measure, we can expect responses to DES items to tell us about how these phenomena are manifested in different populations. Thus just as symptoms of an illness define its parameters, patterns of responses to items and groups of items will, in turn, help define the parameters of dissociation.

To address the definition and measurement of dissociation, we must first address the accuracy of the scale in measuring dissociation. This includes studying both the reliability and the validity of the scale in measuring dissociation. Next, research that informs us about the parameters of dissociation is discussed. Results of research on what construct the DES is measuring turn out to be rather complicated, but they begin to address the issue of how dissociation is currently defined. Research on dissociation in the general population is also described along with some suggestions for how we might understand these results.

Reliability and Validity of the DES

Measurement of any psychological state is an intricate and challenging endeavor, and the reliability and validity of a measure must always be established empirically. This section describes the DES and its administration and scoring and reviews research on the reliability and validity of this scale.

The DES is a 28-item self-report measure of dissociation or the lack of integration of thoughts, feelings, and experiences into the stream of consciousness. Items inquire about the frequency of various experiences of amnestic experiences, gaps in awareness, depersonalization, derealization, absorption, and imaginative involvement (Bernstein and Putnam 1986). Examples of dissociative experiences include having no memory for important past events in your life (amnesia), being in a familiar place and finding it strange and unfamiliar (derealization), feeling that your body does not belong to you (depersonalization), and becoming so absorbed in watching television or a movie that you are unaware of what is happening around you (absorption). Directions on the DES cover sheet specify that subjects should not include experiences that occurred when they were under the influence of alcohol or drugs. The scale takes about 10 minutes to complete and yields item and total scores that range from 0 to 100. A score of 0 means that the subject never has the experience described in the item, and a score of 100 means that the subject always has the experience described in the item. Total scores are calculated by averaging the scores of the 28 items.

Test-retest reliability for the DES has ranged from .84 to .96 in studies with test-retest intervals of 4–6 weeks (Bernstein and Putnam 1986; Frischholz et al. 1990; Pitblado and Sanders 1991). Frischholz et al. (1990) also measured the interrater reliability for scoring of the DES and found a coefficient of absolute agreement of .96. Studies of the internal reliability of the DES have investigated the degree of consistency of item scores across the scale. Split-half reliability studies have divided the DES into two theoretically equivalent halves and then correlated scores on the two halves, yielding split-half reliability correlations ranging from .83 to .93 (Bernstein and Putnam 1986; Pitblado and Sanders 1991). A separate study of internal consistency of the scale calculated the average correlation between test-halves for all possible splits of the test. This yielded a Cronbach's alpha of .95 (Frischholz et al. 1990). High levels of both types of reliability (test-retest and internal) have been found in clinical as well as nonclinical populations (Bernstein and Putnam 1986; Frischholz et al. 1990). In short, the DES has proved to be a very reliable measure.

The validity of a measure can and should be assessed using a broad range of methods. Most importantly, the construct validity of a measure should be studied so that its nature and scope can be empirically established and confirmed. If the scale measures what mental health professionals define as *dissociation,* then those individuals with dissociative disorders (or disorders with a significant dissociative component) should score higher on the scale than those with no disorder or with other nondissociative disorders.

This first aspect of validity has been established and replicated in several studies. As a group, subjects with dissociative identity disorder (DID; the most severe of the dissociative disorders [formerly called multiple personality disorder]) score higher than any other group of subjects (Bernstein and Putnam 1986; Carlson et al. 1993; Frischholz et al. 1990; Ross et al. 1988). The largest and most recent study (Carlson et al. 1993) found a mean DES score of 43 for DID subjects ($N = 228$). Another diagnostic group that has been observed to show high levels of dissociation is that of posttraumatic stress disorder (PTSD) (D. Spiegel et al. 1988). A study including 116

PTSD subjects found a mean DES score of 30 for this group (Carlson et al. 1991). This finding is consistent with results of other studies of PTSD subjects (Branscomb 1991; Bremner et al. 1992; Carlson and Rosser-Hogan 1991). Scores for DID and PTSD subjects were higher than mean scores for any other diagnostic group (including affective, anxiety, neurological, and schizophrenic disorders) and are much higher than DES scores in a non-clinical (general population) sample (N = 523) of 8.6 (Carlson et al. 1993). Clearly, samples of subjects who would be expected to show high levels of dissociation do produce very high DES scores.

Another aspect of validity involves the predictive capacity of the DES. If the DES is a valid measure, it should be able to differentiate between subjects with dissociative disorders and those with other types of disorders. A large multicenter study of the predictive validity of the DES used a cutoff score of 30 to classify a group of 1,051 psychiatric subjects as *DID* or *not DID*. This analysis yielded a sensitivity rate of 74% and a specificity rate of 80% (Carlson et al. 1993). In other words, about three-fourths of those with DID were correctly identified, and over three-fourths of those who were not DID were correctly identified. These results demonstrate good predictive validity for the DES and provide additional evidence that the scale measures what mental health professionals consider dissociation.

What Is Being Measured?

Total DES scores sometimes have different meanings for subjects from different populations. Specifically, contributions to the total DES score of items of varying nature and severity can vary across populations. For example, when DES responses from a nonclinical sample of adults are compared with responses from a sample of psychiatric patients, the nonclinical subjects will tend to endorse fewer DES items and to endorse them at lower rates than do psychiatric patients. This was found to be the case in the original validation study of the DES (Bernstein and Putnam 1986) and has been confirmed in a subsequent large-scale, multicenter study (Carlson et al. 1993). In addition, nonclinical subjects tend to endorse mild forms of dissociation (such as not paying attention to a speaker), whereas psychiatric patients endorse mild dissociative experiences as well as more severe ones (such as lack of memory for important life events). The DES score for a nonclinical subject may reflect less severe experiences of dissociation than those experienced by a psychiatric patient, even if the two subjects have the *same* total DES score.

On the DES, the mild dissociation items tend to be those describing experiences of absorption and imaginative involvement, whereas the most severe items tend to be those describing amnestic experiences. Consequently, DES scores for nonclinical groups tend to reflect experiences of absorption and imaginative involvement, whereas DES scores across a wide spectrum of psychiatric disorders reflect a wide range of dissociative experiences, including such experiences as severe amnesia. It seems then that the answer to the question of what the DES measures varies depending on what population is of interest. In nonclinical populations, the DES may measure absorption and imaginative involvement, whereas in psychiatric populations, it may measure a wider range of dissociative experiences. Because we have long derived our definitions of dissociation from clinical populations, I believe we need to think carefully about the implications of these results. Is a definition of dissociation that is derived from clinical populations and includes more severe dissociation the best one to apply to the general population? Are the kinds of dissociation experienced by non-clinical populations qualitatively as well as quantitatively different from the kinds experienced by psychiatric populations? Should we determine one definition of dissociation to apply to both clinical and nonclinical populations, or should we use different definitions for the different populations? We need to consider these most basic questions if we want to get the most out of future research.

Measuring Dissociation in Nonclinical Populations

Some data are already available that provide information about the incidence of dissociation in the general population. Two fairly large-scale studies have used the DES to measure dissociation in nonclinical populations. Here, the terms *general population* and *nonclinical* are not meant to imply *normal*. These subjects were not specifically identified as having a particular mental disorder, but they were not screened to determine whether any disorder was present. The samples represent a mix of subjects who are predominantly, but not entirely, disorder free.

One study (Carlson et al. 1991) of nonclinical subjects found a mean DES score of 8.6 (N = 573; SD = 10.0). A second study (Ross et al. 1990) that carefully selected a sample of a general population (stratified for race and socioeconomic status) reported a mean DES score of 10.8 (N = 1,055; SD = 10.2). Frequency distributions of the DES scores across the two studies were quite similar. Both were highly positively skewed, with about 85% of the first sample and 80% of the second sample scoring 15 or less on the scale. A small negative correlation between age and DES scores was found in both studies. The explanation for this correlation between age and dissociation scores is not yet clear. There are several possible reasons why younger people score higher on the DES. It may be because they have more dissociative experiences, because they are more willing or prone to report the experiences, or because they are more likely to interpret their experiences as matching those described in the DES items. All three of these possibilities seem likely.

A comparison of the distribution of DES scores across age intervals for men and women showed slightly different patterns for the two sexes. Whereas the DES scores for men seem to decrease gradually across adulthood, reaching a low point in the 50–59 years age interval, DES scores for women seem to fluctuate across the lifespan, reaching low points in the 30–39 years and 50–59 years age intervals. These findings were consistent across both of the nonclinical population studies (Carlson et al. 1991; Ross et al. 1990) and have not yet been explained.

Because subjects from nonclinical populations score in the low range of possible scores on the DES, less differentiation is possible across individuals. Within a nonclinical population, it is not yet clear how meaningful small differences in DES scores across individuals will prove to be. However, because subjects with medical and physical conditions may well score in a wider range than nonclinical subjects, it is possible that meaningful comparisons could be made between those with and without physical and medical conditions. Again, the conclusions we come to from general population data will depend on the definition of dissociation we apply. The meaning of these results in light of a clinically based definition of dissociation will be very different from their meaning in light of an alternative definition of the phenomenon.

HYPNOTIZABILITY AND DISSOCIATION

The DES has been used to study the relationship between hypnotizability and dissociation in a number of studies. Before reviewing these studies, it is important to consider whether we should expect DES scores to be related to scores on standard scales of hypnotizability (e.g., the Stanford Hypnotic Susceptibility Scale [SHSS; Weitzenhoffer and Hilgard 1962] and the Harvard

Group Scale of Hypnotic Susceptibility [HGSHS; Shor and Orne 1962]).

Several authors have noted an apparent relationship between hypnotic susceptibility and dissociation (Frischholz 1985; Hilgard 1986; D. Spiegel et al. 1988). But in a 1989 article by Carlson and Putnam that reviews research in the area in depth, it was noted that standard scales of hypnotizability measure behaviors that are in a different realm from those measured by the DES. Hypnotic susceptibility scales measure alterations in motor, sensory, and cognitive functions, whereas the DES measures alterations in memory, awareness, identity, cognitions, and perceptions. Because the two types of scales sample from different domains, correlations between scores on the two would be reduced or low if individuals' experiences across the domains vary.

The scales also differ greatly in the method used to measure each phe-nomenon and the type of data it provides. Whereas susceptibility scales actually sample an individual's capacity to experience hypnotic phenomena in an experimental or clinical context, the DES obtains self-reports on the frequency of dissociative experiences on a day-to-day basis. The former seem to measure experience on the micro level, whereas the latter measures experience on the macro level. The DES could be described to be measur-ing *dissociativity*. This term would be defined as the tendency to have dissociative experiences on a day-to-day basis.

In addition, the DES tends to measure experiences that are more spon-taneous and involuntary than those measured by hypnotic susceptibility scales (Carlson and Putnam 1989). It is unclear at this time how much measures of hypnotizability can tell us about an individual's experiences of daily, spontaneous alterations in consciousness. It is important that these differences in what is being measured and how it is measured be kept in mind when considering studies comparing DES and hypnotizability scores.

Two recent studies (Nadon et al. 1991; Westergaard et al. 1991) used college students as subjects and correlated scores on the DES and the HGSHS–Form A. The Westergaard study found a correlation of .03 (NS, $N=$ 217) between the two measures, whereas the Nadon et al. study found a correlation of .14 ($P<.05$, $N=475$). In striking contrast are the findings of Campbell Perry (unpublished data, 1986) who correlated scores of college students on the DES and the SHSS–Form C and obtained a correlation of .61 ($P<.0001$, $N=60$). Through a personal communication (C. Perry, March 1987), I have learned that these results have since been replicated on a separate sample of 41 subjects.

One plausible explanation for these discrepant findings across studies lies in the hypnotizability levels of the subjects. In the Perry study, 20 subjects were selected at each of three levels of hypnotizability (low, medium, and high). This method of selection results in an increase in the number of subjects in the low and high categories compared with what would be obtained through random sampling. This alteration in the distribution of hypnotizability scores in the sample has an effect similar to an expansion of the range of hypnotizability scores: It causes an increase in the size of the correlation coefficient. The question that remains is which range gives us the most useful information about the relationship between the two phenomena.

Despite the fact that its sample does not accurately reflect the general population, the Perry study provides very useful and accurate information about the relationship between hypnotizability and dissociation. The mean DES scores for the three levels of hypnotizability in the study were 10.3, 18.5, and 30.8, respectively. Clearly, higher levels of hypnotizability are related to higher DES scores. The question that remains is whether the findings can be applied to a general population.

Imagine for a moment a scatterplot of the Perry data with hypnotizability scores plotted against DES scores. It shows visually the .61 correlation calculated. There are more data points in the lower left and upper right quadrants than there would be if the sample were randomly selected. If one threw out the extra data for a moment and imagined a scatterplot of the same data with 24 subjects removed (12 from the group with low hypnotizability and 12 from the group with high hypnotizability), there would be fewer data points in the lower left and upper right quadrants. The correlation calculated from this reduced set of points would be noticeably lower but the data have not changed. The relationship is still present and strong. Those with the lowest DES scores still tend to have lower hypnotizability scores, and those with the highest DES scores still tend to have higher hypnotizability scores.

What then can we conclude about the relationship between the two phenomena? The results now available indicate that the ability to experience hypnotic phenomena and the tendency to dissociate on a day-to-day basis are related but distinct constructs. Hypnotizability measures may be good predictors of some variables, whereas the DES may be a good predictor of others. There may also be contexts in which both types of measures provide valuable information about the variables of interest. The value of using both types of measures in one of these contexts (the experience of pain) is discussed below.

A clear understanding of the relationship between hypnotizability and dissociation will not come, however, until a great deal more research has been done. One example of an area of investigation that might be fruitful involves examining responses to DES item scores. An examination of average DES item scores across three levels of hypnotizability from the Perry study shows that some of the scores vary little across groups, whereas others vary greatly (C. Perry, unpublished data, 1986). It might be possible to understand more about the overlap in the constructs of hypnotizability and dissociation if the content of the items that vary little and that of the items that vary greatly were analyzed.

Another avenue for research that is just beginning to be explored is the relationship between dissociation, measured by the DES, and hypnotizability, measured by the Hypnotic Induction Profile (HIP; H. Spiegel 1974). The HIP is a brief measure of hypnotic responsivity that was developed as an alternative to the more lengthy standard measures. The HIP is similar to standard scales of hypnotizability (SHSS–Forms A and C) in that correlations between scores on the measures are moderate and statistically significant (Frischholz et al. 1987). It differs from standard scales and is similar to the DES in that items inquire about the subjective experience of dissociation and involuntariness. In addition, scores on the HIP have been found to correlate moderately and significantly with scores on the Tellegen Absorption Scale (Tellegen and Atkinson 1974), a measure of the tendency to become absorbed in experiences and activities. Because the HIP is a measure of hypnotizability that samples from the same domain as the DES, and because it has been found to correlate well with another related dispositional measure, it seems likely that exploration of the relationship between the DES and the HIP will provide new information about the relationship between dissociation and hypnotizability. Other avenues for research that might be useful have been described elsewhere (Carlson and Putnam 1989), and still more are suggested in other chapters in this book.

MEASURING DISSOCIATION IN RELATION TO PHYSICAL AND MEDICAL CONDITIONS

Availability of the DES as a simple method of studying dissociation in subjects with various somatic disorders or conditions opens up a wealth of interesting research questions. Many of these questions relate directly to issues of mind-body interaction and to the possibilities of psychological control over bodily sensations. The latter area of study has been dominated in the past by research on the properties of hypnosis and the abilities of hypnotic subjects to modify their experience of physical sensations. The use of hypnosis certainly has a profound impact on the treatment of physical disorders. But measures of hypnotizability may tell us little about spontaneously occurring alterations in consciousness. Availability of a convenient measure of dissociation allows us to ask questions about the relationships between somatic states and spontaneous alterations in consciousness.

Research findings from studies that measured dissociation in relation to a wide variety of somatic conditions have recently become available. Conditions studied include seizure disorders, premenstrual syndrome, eating disorders, and physical and sexual abuse. Some very interesting research on the relationship between DES scores and the ability to tolerate pain has also recently been completed.

Seizure Disorders

There have been a number of case studies in clinical literature reporting dissociative symptoms in seizure disorder patients (see Devinsky et al. 1989 and Loewenstein and Putnam 1988 for review of this literature). A few authors have suggested that neurological abnormalities present in seizure disorders may be the cause of dissociative symptoms. If this were the case, patients with seizure disorders should show high levels of dissociative symptomatology. To investigate this possibility, two studies (Devinsky et al. 1989; Loewenstein and Putnam 1988) have used the DES to measure dissociation in seizure patients. In both studies, patients being treated or evaluated for seizure disorders (including complex seizures, generalized seizures, or both) were given the DES. In one of these studies (Loewenstein and Putnam 1988), the mean length of illness was 10.4 years and the mean frequency of seizures (all types) was just over four times per week. Results of both studies show that seizure patients produce scores on the DES that are comparable to those of control subjects. These findings contradict the hypothesis that the neurological abnormalities associated with seizures are responsible for dissociative experiences, and it seems reasonable to accept this conclusion until results of any empirical study show otherwise. Nevertheless, dissociative symptoms may still be mistaken for seizures, and the DES may be useful in distinguishing highly dissociative patients from patients with seizure disorders.

Premenstrual Syndrome

Evidence of a link between a physiological process and dissociation has been found in a study of menstrual cycle changes in women with premenstrual syndrome (PMS) (Jensvold et al. 1989). Dissociative symptoms were measured with the DES in 42 stringently diagnosed PMS patients and 38 control subjects. DES scores obtained during follicular and luteal phases were compared in patient and control groups. Results showed higher levels of dissociation in both luteal and follicular phases for PMS subjects compared with control subjects. Further, whereas control subjects showed no change in level of dissociation across the two phases, PMS subjects showed elevated DES scores during the luteal phase. This elevation may be due to hormonal changes or related to increased levels of pain during this phase. Although the finding of psychological changes occurring during the luteal phase is not new, the elevated dissociation level for PMS subjects during the follicular phase is intriguing.

Further research may lead to increased understanding of PMS and may shed light on the physiological mechanisms involved with dissociation. Does PMS have a primarily physiological origin, a primarily psychological origin, or are there individual differences in the etiology of the disorder? Is there an underlying physiological predisposition for the disorder that is potentiated by particular psychological stresses? Is increased dissociation in PMS patients a response to increased experience of pain, or are both dissociation and the increased pain caused by some third variable? The DES could be used to study these and other intriguing questions about PMS.

Eating Disorders

Case reports of dissociative symptoms and findings of high levels of hypnotizability in patients with eating disorders led Demitrack et al. (1990) to investigate dissociation levels in anorexic and bulimic subjects. They found that both groups produced substantially higher overall DES scores compared with a group of age- and sex-matched control subjects. The median score for the bulimic group (16.6) was more than twice as high as the median score for the control group (6.4), whereas the median score for the anorexic group (19.5) was about three times that of the control group. In light of their findings, the authors suggest that neurochemical abnormalities in patients with eating disorders may provide information about the physiological underpinnings of dissociative experiences (Demitrack et al. 1990).

Because eating disorders are frequently reported to occur in patients with histories of childhood sexual abuse, it is worth considering whether abuse experiences of subjects with eating disorders might be leading to higher dissociation scores. The connection between eating disorders and past abuse appears to be a complicated and controversial issue, however. Two recent reviews (Coovert et al. 1989; Pope and Hudson 1992) of the literature in this area have concluded that controlled studies have generally not found that patients with eating disorders show a higher prevalence of childhood sexual abuse than control subjects or than general population subjects. In light of these findings, it seems likely that some factor other than abuse history must be found to account for high levels of dissociation in subjects with eating disorders.

Physical and Sexual Abuse

Several researchers have begun to study the relationship between experiences of past physical and sexual abuse and dissociative symptoms. Although this area of study does not focus on a physical condition per se, the somatic aspects of childhood experiences of physical and sexual abuse make it likely that research on this population will produce useful information about the link between physical states and dissociative experiences. In particular, this research may provide insight into the question of how dissociation functions to maintain mental and physical homeostasis during episodes of physical and sexual abuse.

Sanders studied the relationship between DES scores and the level of unpredictable violence that college student subjects reported experiencing during childhood (Sanders et al. 1989). Sanders asked subjects about the level of unpredictable violence in their homes when they were growing up. She compared DES scores across three levels of reported unpredictable violence during childhood (subjects answered "not at all," "somewhat," or "very much") and found a significant difference in DES scores across groups. Subjects who reported experiencing greater frequency of unpredictable violence also scored higher on the DES.

Chu and Dill (1990) studied the relationship between sexual abuse history and DES scores in female psychiatric inpatients. Those with histories of physical abuse scored higher than those without such histories, and those with histories of sexual abuse scored higher than those without such histories. Subjects with histories of both physical and sexual abuse scored higher than subjects in any other group. The average DES score for subjects who suffered both types of abuse was similar to that found in PTSD patients. In addition, the relationship of the abuser to the subject was found to be an important variable in that subjects who were abused by family members were more dissociative than those abused by someone other than a family member.

Another study in this area explored the relationship between levels of dissociation and two additional abuse variables in psychiatric inpatients. Kirby et al. (1993) have found a positive relationship between severity of childhood abuse and DES scores and between frequency of childhood abuse experiences and DES scores. In addition, a negative relationship was found between the age at onset of abuse and DES scores. It appears, then, that adults who experienced abuse that was more severe, was more frequent, and began earlier all show higher levels of dissociation as adults. A likely interpretation of these findings is that dissociation is an adaptive state change for children during abuse that becomes maladaptive when used chronically as an adult (Putnam 1985). This type of research will no doubt be valuable to those studying the use of dissociation by children to protect against physical and emotional pain.

Pain

One final study of a physical condition that has produced intriguing results is a study of the relationship between pain (produced by the constant pressure of a blood-pressure cuff) and level of dissociation as measured by the DES. A study of 96 subjects compared those who scored above 20 on the DES with those who scored below 20 in terms of how long they tolerated the pain produced by the cuff. Results showed that the high-scoring DES subjects stayed in the cuff significantly longer than the low-scoring DES subjects ($F = 7.6$; df = 1,95; $P < .007$). The high DES subjects stayed in the cuff an average of 9.8 minutes (SD = 5.1), whereas the low DES subjects stayed in the cuff an average of 7.3 minutes (SD = 3.9; Giolas and Sanders 1992).

Perhaps even more interesting was an additional finding of this study involving the relationship between DES scores and the subjective experience of suffering during the procedure. A small, statistically significant correlation was found between these two variables (Pearson's $r = -.20$, $P < .05$), indicating that those with higher DES scores felt they suffered less than those with low DES scores (Giolas and Sanders 1992). It will be interesting to see if these findings can be replicated and whether they will generalize beyond the lab to medical settings. It will also be important to determine how the DES compares with hypnotizability measures as a means of understanding or predicting the relationship between pain and suffering.

USE OF THE DISSOCIATIVE EXPERIENCES SCALE IN TRANSLATION

The DES has been translated for use in several other languages, including French, Spanish, Italian, Dutch, Hindi, Cambodian, Hebrew, Japanese, Swedish, Norwegian, and Czech. Translation is currently in progress for a German version. Much research using the DES in translation is in progress at present, but little has been published to date in English language journals. One published study compares scores of Dutch and American dissociative and general population subjects (Ensink and van Otterloo 1989). In this study, Dutch college students scored somewhat higher than American college student samples, but DID patients scored similarly (Ensink and van Otterloo 1989). The DES was also used in translation to measure levels of dissociation in Cambodian refugees living in the United States (Carlson and Rosser-Hogan 1991). Results of that study showed that refugees' scores were similar to those of U.S. subjects with PTSD. As further studies are published, it will be interesting to see what role culture plays in experiences of dissociation. The extent to which the concept of dissociation can be applied across cultures will be important to those investigating the relationship between physical and psychological states in other countries as well as to those studying these issues in ethnic subcultures in the United States.

There are several important issues to be aware of when translating psychological measures across languages and cultures. Some useful guidelines for translation of research instruments are provided by Brislin (1986). Four of the most important issues will be described briefly here. First, it is important to translate items conceptually and not literally. This method ensures that colloquial expressions are not translated literally and that terms and concepts unfamiliar in another culture do not appear in the translated items. Second, it is sometimes necessary to eliminate items that do not make sense conceptually in another culture or population. For example, in translating symptoms for PTSD, it would have been meaningless to ask refugees if they had lost interest in their usual activities after a traumatic experience. Because the subjects were unable to engage in any of their previous activities in Cambodia, it was considered wise to eliminate this item (Carlson and Rosser-Hogan 1991). Third, it is likewise important to include new items that represent experiences that do occur in the second culture but were not part of the cultural experience of those for whom the measure was originally developed (A. Kleinman, personal communication, October 1991). Fourth, it is crucial to perform a blind backtranslation of the translated measure so that the backtranslation can be compared and reconciled with the original version. This process provides a necessary check on the accuracy of the translation.

CONCLUSION

In conclusion, this chapter provides more questions than answers about the relationships among dissociation, other psychological states, and physical conditions. Future areas of research that might be fruitful include the question of whether dissociation is a natural response to chronic physical pain. A better understanding of psychological responses to physical pain may lead to new ways to treat patients with chronic pain. A related research question is whether dissociation (or particular types of dissociation) might be used as a predictor of patients' abilities to influence their own physiological processes, such as the experience of pain and the efficiency of immune function. DES scores (or subscale scores) might be useful in predicting which patients would be most successful in using techniques such as hypnosis or imaging to control chronic pain or boost immune functions. It may also be possible to train patients to be more effective in their control of physiological processes. If this were the case, DES scores (or subscores) could be used to identify patients in need of training and to gauge progress in acquisition of imaging or hypnotic skills.

Clearly, there are a wide range of physiological processes and somatic conditions that could be studied using the DES. Research to date has only scratched the surface of possible areas of investigation. Fortunately, tools now are available to accurately measure dissociation. Results of research to date indicate that the DES is a reliable, valid, convenient, and cost-effective measure of day-to-day experiences of dissociation. Several studies have replicated initial findings at independent sites, and findings from studies of a variety of populations and conditions have produced results consistent with predictions. In addition, those interested in studying these same issues in children and adolescents can make use of dissociation scales designed specifically for these populations. The Child Dissociative Checklist (CDC) is a reliable and valid measure that can be used to study dissociation in children (Putnam et al., in press), and the Adolescent DES is now being developed by the authors of the DES for use with adolescents. These self-report measures are sure to be valuable tools in future research on the interaction between physical and psychological states.

REFERENCES

Bernstein EM, Putnam FW: Development, reliability, and validity of a dissociation scale. J Nerv Ment Dis 174:727–735, 1986

Branscomb L: Dissociation in combat-related post-traumatic stress disorder. Dissociation 4:13–20, 1991

Bremner JD, Southwick S, Brett E, et al: Dissociation and posttraumatic stress disorder in Vietnam combat veterans. Am J Psychiatry 149:328–333, 1992

Brislin R: The wording and translation of research instruments, in Field Methods in Cross-Cultural Research. Edited by Lonner WJ, Berry JW. Newbury Park, CA, Sage, 1986, pp 137–164

Carlson EB, Putnam FW: Integrating research in dissociation and hypnotic susceptibility: are there two pathways to hypnotizability? Dissociation 2:32–38, 1989

Carlson EB, Putnam FW, Ross CA, et al: Factor analysis of the Dissociative Experiences Scale: a multicenter study. Paper presented at the Eighth International Conference on Multiple Personality and Dissociative States, Chicago, IL, November 1991

Carlson EB, Putnam FW, Ross CA, et al: Validity of the Dissociative Experiences Scale in screening for multiple personality disorder: a multicenter study. Am J Psychiatry 150:1030–1036, 1993

Carlson EB, Rosser-Hogan R: Trauma experiences, posttraumatic stress, dissociation, and depression in Cambodian refugees. Am J Psychiatry 148:1548–1551, 1991

Chu JA, Dill DL: Dissociation in relation to childhood physical and sexual abuse. Am J Psychiatry 147:887–892, 1990

Coovert DL, Kinder BN, Thompson JK: The psychosexual aspects of anorexia nervosa and bulimia nervosa: a review of the literature. Clinical Psychology Review 9:169–180, 1989

Demitrack MA, Putnam FW, Brewerton TD, et al: Relation of clinical variables to dissociative phenomena in eating disorders. Am J Psychiatry 147:1184–1188, 1990

Devinsky O, Putnam FW, Grafman J, et al: Dissociative states and epilepsy. Neurology 39:835–840, 1989

Ensink BJ, van Otterloo D: A validation of the Dissociative Experiences Scale in the Netherlands. Dissociation 2:221–223, 1989

Frischholz EJ: The relationship among dissociation, hypnosis, and child abuse in the development of multiple personality disorder, in Childhood Antecedents of Multiple Personality Disorder. Edited by Kluft RP. Washington, DC, American Psychiatric Press, 1985, pp 110–126

Frischholz EJ, Braun BG, Sachs RG, et al: The Dissociative Experiences Scale: further replication and validation. Dissociation 3:151–153, 1990

Frischholz EJ, Spiegel DA, Trentalange MJ, et al: The Hypnotic Induction Profile and absorption. Am J Clin Hypn 30:87–93, 1987

Giolas MH, Sanders B: Pain and suffering as a function of dissociation level and instructional set. Dissociation 5:205–209, 1992

Hilgard ER: Divided Consciousness: Multiple Controls in Human Thought and Action. New York, Wiley, 1986

Jensvold M, Putnam FW, Schmidt P, et al: Abuse, dissociation, and posttraumatic stress disorder in premenstrual syndrome patients and controls. Paper presented at the Sixth International Conference on Multiple Personality and Dissociative States, Chicago, IL, November 1989

Kirby JS, Chu JA, Dill DL: Correlates of dissociative symptomatology in patients with physical and sexual abuse histories. Compr Psychiatry 34:258–263, 1993

Loewenstein RJ, Putnam FW: A comparison study of dissociative symptoms in patients with complex partial seizures, multiple personality disorder, and posttraumatic stress disorder. Dissociation 1:17–23, 1988

Nadon R, Hoyt IP, Register PA, et al: Absorption and hypnotizability: context effects reexamined. J Pers Soc Psychol 60:144–153, 1991

Pitblado CB, Sanders B: Reliability and short-term stability of scores on the Dissociative Experiences Scale. Paper presented at the Eighth International Conference on Multiple Personality and Dissociative States, Chicago, IL, November 1991

Pope HG, Hudson JI: Is childhood sexual abuse a risk factor for bulimia nervosa? Am J Psychiatry 149:455–463, 1992

Putnam FW Jr: Dissociation as a response to extreme trauma, in Childhood Antecedents of Multiple Personality. Edited by Kluft RP. Washington, DC, American Psychiatric Press, 1985, pp 65–97

Putnam FW Jr, Helmers K, Trickett PK: Development, reliability, and validity of a child dissociation scale. Child Abuse and Neglect (in press)

Ross CA, Joshi S, Currie R: Dissociation experiences in the general population. Am J Psychiatry 147:1547–1552, 1990

Ross CA, Norton GR, Anderson G: The Dissociative Experiences Scale: a replication study. Dissociation 1:21–22, 1988

Sanders B, McRoberts G, Tollefson C: Childhood stress and dissociation in a college population. Dissociation 2:17–23, 1989

Shor RE, Orne E: Harvard Group Scale of Hypnotic Susceptibility. Palo Alto, CA, Consulting Psychologists Press, 1962

Spiegel D, Hunt T, Dondershine HF: Dissociation and hypnotizability in posttraumatic stress disorder. Am J Psychiatry 145:301–305, 1988

Spiegel H: Eye-Roll Levitation Method: Manual for the Hypnotic Induction Profile. New York, Soni Media, 1974

Tellegen A, Atkinson G: Openness to absorbing and self-altering experiences ("absorption"), a trait related to hypnotic susceptibility. J Abnorm Psychol 83:268–277, 1974

Weitzenhoffer AM, Hilgard ER: Stanford Hypnotic Susceptibility Scale. Palo Alto, CA, Consulting Psychologists Press, 1962

Westergaard C, Frischholz EJ, Braun BG, et al: The relation between the Dissociative Experiences Scale and hypnotizability. Paper presented at the Eighth International Conference on Multiple Personality and Dissociative States, Chicago, IL, November 1991

CHAPTER 4

Systematizing Dissociation: Symptomatology and Diagnostic Assessment

Marlene Steinberg, M.D.

HISTORICAL OVERVIEW

Dissociation has been observed throughout human history (Quen 1986). Theoretical conceptualizations of dissociation date in some instances from the origin of modern psychiatric inquiry (Ellenberger 1970). Many pioneers of the field interpreted dissociation in the context of rival theories of mind; philosophical, religious, biological, and cognitive pictures of human consciousness; and maps of subconscious, unconscious, or coconscious processes (Freud 1915/1963; Hart 1910, 1926; Münsterberg 1907; F. Myers 1903; Prince 1907; Sidis 1911). Contemporary reviews relate dissociation to a variety of phenomena, including habitual and automatic activities, parallel processing, neuropsychophysiologic state-dependent learning, and divisions between executive and monitoring functions or between mental rep-

This research was supported by NIMH First Independent Research Support and Transition Award MH43352. I thank David Spiegel, M.D., and John Kihlstrom, Ph.D., for their comments on an earlier draft. Portions of this chapter were presented as an invited address, titled "The Structured Clinical Interview for DSM-III-R Dissociative Disorders" on October 18, 1991, at the Dissociation Workshop for the Research Network on Mind-Body Interactions, sponsored by the John D. and Catherine T. MacArthur Foundation in Menlo Park, California.

resentations of the self and representations of experience, thought, and action (Braun 1984; Hilgard 1986; Kihlstrom 1987; Kihlstrom and Hoyt 1990). Investigators have noted similarities between clinical dissociation and hypnotic states but differ in their interpretation of the relationship between these phenomena (Bowers 1990; Hilgard 1986; Kihlstrom and Hoyt 1990; D. Spiegel 1990; H. Spiegel and D. Spiegel 1987). There is a range of viewpoints about the compatibility of theories of dissociation and repression (Erdelyi 1985; Singer and Sincoff 1990).

DEFINING DISSOCIATION

Despite the controversy about the theoretical processes underlying dissociative phenomena, there appears to be essential agreement among scholars about the overall phenomenology of dissociation. Nemiah (1991) describes *dissociation* as "the exclusion from consciousness and the inaccessibility of voluntary recall of mental events, singly or in clusters, of varying degrees of complexity, such as memories, sensations, feelings, fantasies, and attitudes." Maintained in an unconscious state, these mental events may intrude into consciousness spontaneously or affect consciousness in the form of ego-alien symptoms. *Dissociation* is defined by Spiegel and Cardeña (1991) as "a structured separation of mental processes (e.g., thoughts, emotions, conation, memory, and identity) that are ordinarily integrated." DSM-IV (American Psychiatric Press 1994) defines the essential features of dissociative disorders as a "disruption in the usually integrated functions of consciousness, memory, identity, or perception of the environment" (p. 477).

Frankel (1990) has argued that these definitions are overly broad. However, any lack of clarity may result from the complexity of the dissociative phenomenon itself, which can best be understood as multidimensional. For clinical purposes, therefore, it is useful to consider the global concept of dissociation in terms of interdependent but discrete components.

ORGANIZING DISSOCIATION:
FIVE MEASURABLE COMPONENTS

To assess dissociative symptoms and disorders, I and colleagues (Steinberg et al. 1990) organized the global definitions of dissociation into five core dissociative symptoms: amnesia, depersonalization, derealization, identity confusion, and identity alteration (see also Steinberg 1993a; Steinberg et al. 1990). Although these five symptoms coexist with a variety of psychiatric disorders, the profiles of these symptoms in patients with dissociative disorders show key distinguishing features (Steinberg 1993b). In this chapter, I briefly review each of the five symptoms and describe the assessment of these symptoms using the Structured Clinical Interview for DSM-IV Dissociative Disorders (SCID-D; Steinberg 1985, 1993a). I also review findings on the reliability and discriminant validity of these instruments. Then, using this conceptualization of dissociative phenomena, I describe the assessment of the dissociative disorders and posttraumatic stress disorder (PTSD).

Amnesia

Amnesia may be defined as the absence from memory of a specific and significant segment of time (Steinberg 1993a; Steinberg et al. 1990). Amnesia can be categorized by etiology and context. *Functional* memory loss can be distinguished from *ordinary forgetting* on the one hand and *organic* amnesia on the other (Schacter and Kihlstrom 1989). Dissociative amnesia falls into the functional category and may be conceptualized in a variety of ways.

Schacter and Kihlstrom (1989) subdivide functional amnesia into amnesias that have *pathological* and *nonpathological* etiologies. Nonpathological amnesias include childhood amnesia, sleep and dream amnesia, and hypnotic amnesia. Pathological amnesias include *functional retrograde amnesia*, which entails loss of personal identity and large sectors of one's personal past; this may be characteristic of dissociative fugue. Patients with dissociative identity disorder (DID; formerly called multiple personality disorder) also commonly experience amnesia between personalities.

As classified in DSM-IV, there are four types of pathological amnesia: *selective amnesia*, which is a failure to recall some events from a circumscribed period; *localized amnesia*, which involves complete failure to recall the events of a circumscribed period of time; *continuous amnesia*, which is a failure to recall events from a specific time up to the present; and *generalized amnesia*, which consists of a loss of memory for one's entire life. Patients with amnestic episodes of psychogenic origin often experience a variety of perceptual alterations in the experience of time, such as the feeling that time is discontinuous.

Dissociative amnesia is regularly encountered in hospital emergency rooms (Nemiah 1985). An investigation of 1,795 consecutive psychiatric admissions to Wright Patterson Air Force Medical Center from 1968 to 1970 revealed that 1.3% of all patients had experienced amnesia (Kirshner 1973). Another report estimates that 20% of all hospital admissions for amnesia are of psychogenic (dissociative) origin (Kiersch 1962).

Depersonalization

Depersonalization is described in the literature as a sense of detachment from the self. Salient features include a feeling of unreality or strangeness of the self, a sense that one is observing the self from outside, and a loss of all affective response except for the unpleasant quality of the symptom (Ackner 1954; Edwards and Angus 1972; Fewtrell 1986; Galdston 1947; Levy and Wachtel 1978; Mayer-Gross 1935; Saperstein 1949; Steinberg 1991, 1993b). A characteristic feature of depersonalization is that reality testing remains intact; the subject will describe his or her estrangement in "as if" terms rather than in terms of an actual detachment or division of the self (Ackner 1954; Fewtrell 1986; Saperstein 1949).

There are a variety of manifestations of depersonalization, including disturbances in identity, such as feeling as if the real self is far away, a feeling of strangeness or unreality of the self, a sense of physical fragmentation or separation from part of one's body, and disturbances in affect, such as an absence of feeling, a feeling of numbness or disconnection from one's emotions, a feeling of being dead, or as if one is an automaton.

Depersonalization is the third most common complaint among psychiatric patients, preceded by anxiety and depression (Cattell 1975). Transient depersonalization syndrome has been noted in close to 40% of inpatients and 30% of patients exposed to life-threatening danger (Noyes and Kletti 1977). Brauer et al. (1970) note that 12% of all psychiatric patients experience severe and lasting depersonalization.

Derealization

Derealization is defined as a sense that one's surroundings are unreal. Derealization may involve a feeling that one's home or workplace is unfamiliar, or a sense that friends or relatives are strange, unfamiliar, or unreal. Although derealization frequently coexists with amnesia, it should be distinguished from amnestic episodes. Although some classify derealization as a disturbance of recognition (Reed 1988), the absence of a familiar affect usually associated with a particular object or person may be the salient factor (Siomopoulos 1972). A patient with derealization may feel that his or her friends or environment are unreal or unfamiliar or find it difficult to recognize family members, yet still be aware of his or her actual identity and history. An individual with derealization may also experience distortions in his or her perception of space or time.

Identity Confusion and Identity Alteration

Definitions and severity ratings of identity confusion and identity alteration were developed specifically for systematic assessment (Steinberg 1993a; Steinberg et al. 1990). *Identity confusion* was defined as a subjective feeling of uncertainty, puzzlement, or conflict about one's own identity. In contrast, *identity alteration* consists of objective behavior indicating the assumption of different identities (Steinberg 1993a, 1993b; Steinberg et al. 1990). Identity alteration may be manifested by a variety of behavioral patterns, including the use of different names, the observation that one possesses a learned skill for which one cannot account, and the discovery of items in one's possession that one is unaware of having acquired.

ASSESSING DISSOCIATION

Difficulties in Assessment

Varied presentations. Dissociative symptoms have often been difficult to detect (Coons 1984; Davison 1964; Edwards and Angus 1972; Kluft 1984b, 1988, 1991; Nemiah 1985; Putnam et al. 1986; Ross and Norton 1988; D. Spiegel 1991). It may be difficult for a subject whose major defense is dissociation to volunteer an accurate history; some subjects will be amnestic for their symptoms, whereas others will seek to hide problems with identity or episodes of depersonalization (Davison 1964; Kluft 1988, 1991; D. Spiegel 1991; Steinberg 1991). Dissociation is rarely the presenting complaint. The varied presentations of dissociative symptoms mimic a spectrum of psychiatric conditions, including psychotic, affective, and character disorders, such as borderline personality disorder, thus complicating assessment (Akhtar and Brenner 1979; Coons et al. 1988; Fink and Golinkoff 1990; Horevitz and Braun 1984; Kluft 1988, 1991; Loewenstein 1991; Nemiah

1985; Putnam et al. 1986; Ross and Norton 1988; Schultz et al. 1989; Steinberg 1991). Investigators report that dissociative symptoms and the dissociative disorders may be more common than originally believed (Bliss and Jeppsen 1985; Coons et al. 1988; Fink and Golinkoff 1990; Horevitz and Braun 1984; Kluft 1988, 1991; Putnam et al. 1986; Ross and Norton 1988; Schultz et al. 1989; Steinberg 1991). Estimates of rates in clinical and community populations vary. Their accuracy has been limited heretofore by the lack of diagnostic tools for dissociative symptoms and the dissociative disorders. The recent development of screening (Bernstein and Putnam 1986; Riley 1988; Sanders 1986) and diagnostic instruments (Ross et al. 1989; Steinberg 1985, 1993a) should facilitate systematic investigation of the incidence and prevalence of dissociative symptoms and the dissociative disorders.

Dissociation and trauma. Research indicates that dissociative symptoms are posttraumatic (Coons et al. 1989; Fine 1990; D. Spiegel 1991; Terr 1991). The close connection between dissociation and severe trauma, child abuse, or incest may complicate assessment because patients may deny or be amnestic for these stressors (Frishholz 1985; Goodwin 1985, 1988; Kirshner 1973; Kluft 1984a, 1991; D. Spiegel 1984, 1991). Studies have noted histories of abuse in 72%–98% of all reported cases of the dissociative disorders (Kluft 1988, 1991; Putnam et al. 1986) and 50%–75% of general psychiatric patients (Bryer et al. 1987; Ellerstein 1980; Emslie and Rosenfelt 1983; Husain and Chapel 1983; M. Myers 1991; Rosenfeld 1979; Sansonnet-Hayden et al. 1987). In a sample of 468 male and female clinical subjects who reported childhood sexual abuse, 59.6% were amnestic for the abuse at some point in their lives (Briere and Conte 1989). Where a history of abuse remains hidden, there is less likelihood that efforts will be made to uncover posttraumatic symptoms. Finally, failure to diagnose these symptoms will, per force, greatly decrease the likelihood that the patient will receive effective treatment (Kluft 1984a, 1985).

The SCID-D

A semistructured diagnostic interview. The SCID-D is a semistructured diagnostic interview developed to systematically assess the presence, severity, and phenomenology of the five posttraumatic dissociative symptoms in patients with all psychiatric disorders and to make DSM-IV diagnoses in the five dissociative disorders (Steinberg 1993a, 1993b; Steinberg et al. 1990). The SCID-D can also be used to assess dissociative symptoms in individuals without psychiatric illness. The five posttraumatic dissociative symptoms assessed in the SCID-D are amnesia, depersonalization, derealization, identity confusion, and identity alteration. The SCID-D is the only diagnostic tool available that assesses the severity of dissociative symptoms and diagnoses dissociative disorders. Modeled on the format of the Structured Clinical Interview for DSM-III-R (SCID), developed by Spitzer et al. (1990), the SCID-D enables the interviewer to make diagnoses in the dissociative disorders on the basis of DSM-IV criteria. Embedded in the interview are the DSM-IV criteria for dissociative amnesia (formerly called psychogenic amnesia), dissociative fugue (formerly called psychogenic fugue), depersonalization disorder, DID, and dissociative disorder not otherwise specified (DDNOS). Questions are designed to elicit responses detailing the full spectrum of each symptom, such as its multifaceted manifestations and information necessary to assess severity (i.e., chronicity, distress, and dysfunction associated with the symptoms). Associated features of dissociative symptoms assessed in the SCID-D include rapid shifts in mood, symptoms, or level of functioning; spontaneous age regressions; traumatic flashbacks; hallucinations; and ongoing internal dialogues.

The SCID-D interview is designed to overcome the difficulty of detecting dissociative symptoms and disorders. Each question is phrased in an open-ended manner, enabling the interviewer to make use of a subject's own descriptions and terminology and reducing the possibility of false negatives and false positives, including malingering. The SCID-D allows a trained clinician to incorporate individualized follow-up questions to explore each positive response. In addition, the interviewer can choose two of nine follow-up sections that further explore previously reported dissociative symptoms for underlying clues of identity alteration. Both direct and indirect questions are used to investigate different aspects of these multifaceted symptoms. Because patients may be amnestic for dissociative symptoms, questions about behavioral manifestations include information that the patient may have learned from friends or family members and the discovery of objects, abilities, or skills associated with an alter identity. Intra-interview dissociative cues are also assessed in order to augment the information verbalized by the patient and to approximate a clinical diagnostic interview.

The SCID-D contains no direct questions about trauma. Rather, it asks about the dissociative defenses that enabled the individual to survive traumatic experiences. However, through open-ended, nonthreatening investigation of posttraumatic symptomatology, the SCID-D often spontaneously elicits a history of traumatic experiences closely related to the symptoms in question.

Guidelines for the administration, interpretation, and scoring of the SCID-D are presented in the *Interviewer's Guide to the SCID-D* (Steinberg 1993b). The *Interviewer's Guide* provides *Severity Rating Definitions* for the scoring of the severity of individual dissociative symptoms. The *Diagnostic Work Sheets* facilitate the systematic diagnosis of DSM-IV dissociative disorders based on numerous cross-referenced SCID-D items.

Reliability and validity studies. Good to excellent reliability and discriminant validity for the SCID-D have been noted (Steinberg 1989–1992; Steinberg et al. 1990). These results have been replicated by Goff et al. (1992) at Harvard and by Boon and Draijer (1991) in Amsterdam. In addition, multicenter field trials of the SCID-D have been completed, and preliminary analysis of the results indicates good to excellent reliability and validity (Steinberg et al. 1989–1993).

In the initial pilot study, the SCID-D was administered to 48 patients with a variety of clinical diagnoses (Steinberg et al. 1986; Steinberg et al. 1990). All interviews were scored independently by a corater who was blind to all of the referring clinicians' diagnoses of the patients. Interexaminer reliability levels of individual SCID-D responses, in terms of total overall assessment, presence or absence of a dissociative disorder, type of dissociative disorder, and specific dissociative symptoms, produced values in the good to excellent range of clinical significance according to the statistical guidelines of Cicchetti and Sparrow (1981) and Fleiss (1981). Data analysis for discriminant validity compared subjects previously diagnosed as having a dissociative disorder, subjects diagnosed with a nondissociative disorder, and normal control subjects. The SCID-D was able to discriminate successfully among these groups of subjects, with experiment-wise error controlled at .05.

As a result of the pilot testing of the SCID-D, I was awarded the first National Institute of Mental Health (NIMH) research grant given to a diagnostic tool for detecting dissociation (Steinberg 1989–1992). The 3-year, NIMH-funded field trials involved the administration and statistical analysis of over 350 SCID-D interviews. Subjects were interviewed twice within 1 week by two of five interviewers blind to referring clinicians' diagnoses. Preliminary analysis of the first 100 subjects with dissociative and nondissociative disorders indicates good to excellent test-retest reliability for each of the five dissociative symptoms and disorders, as well as discriminant validity among different populations.

Several other investigations of the reliability and validity of the SCID-D are in progress, including a multicenter study with experts in the field at four sites in the United States (Steinberg et al. 1989–1993) and a cross-national replication and expansion study in Amsterdam. Preliminary results of the Dutch study indicate good to excellent reliability and validity for the dissociative symptoms and the dissociative disorders (Boon and Draijer 1991). The phenomenology of each of the five dissociative symptoms for Dutch subjects was virtually identical to results obtained in the Unites States, as were the constellations of symptoms manifesting for each dissociative disorder.

Assessing the Five Dissociative Symptoms

In order to evaluate dissociative symptoms, as with other psychiatric symptoms, it is necessary to assess the nature, frequency, and duration of episodes; the impairment of functioning; and the presence or absence of precipitating stressors. The Severity Rating Definitions developed for the SCID-D evaluate symptom severity in terms of these features. After the interview, each symptom receives the following overall ratings, which are numerically coded: none (1), mild (2), moderate (3), or severe (4). These ratings combine for a total SCID-D score that ranges from 5 (no dissociative symptoms) to 20 (very severe symptoms). For an example of the severity rating definitions, see the definitions for depersonalization in Table 4–1.

Assessing amnesia.　Of the five dissociative symptoms, amnesia is often the most difficult to assess. Because amnesia represents an absence of memory, patients may be unaware that something is missing from their memory. In other words, patients can be amnestic for their amnesia (Kluft 1988). It is often difficult to obtain a reliable estimate from the patients of the frequency of their amnestic episodes, as patients with the most chronic amnesia often have learned to adapt to, or compensate for, their amnesia. Clinically, histories of amnesia may be described in terms of blank spells, "blacking out" or "spacing out," in the absence of temporal lobe epilepsy or other organic etiology. Individuals with chronic amnesia often confabulate replies in an attempt to fill gaps in memory. During the SCID-D interview, a pattern of vagueness or inconsistency in answering questions may indicate amnesia in an otherwise cooperative patient. Sudden disorientation during the course of an interview may also indicate the symptom of amnesia.

Other indications include a history of finding oneself in a place and not knowing how or why one arrived there, finding unfamiliar objects in one's possession, disavowing actions that are confirmed by observers, and a history at any time of having lost one's identity.

The SCID-D is structured to approach amnesia both directly and indirectly. The first question dealing with amnesia, question 1, "Have you ever felt as if there were large gaps in your memory?," is followed by questions tapping into further amnesia and identity confusion, such as question 11,

Table 4–1.   Severity Rating Definitions of individual dissociative symptoms

Depersonalization—Detachment from oneself (e.g., a sense of looking at oneself as if one is an outsider)	**SCID-D items**
Mild	
● Single episode or rare (total of 1–4) episodes of depersonalization that are brief (less than 4 hours) and are usually associated with stress or fatigue.	38–47, 54, 55, 64
Moderate (one of the following)	
● Recurrent (more than 4) episodes of depersonalization. (May be brief or prolonged. May be precipitated by stress.)	38–47, 54, 55, 64
● Episodes (1–4) of depersonalization that (one of the following)	
● Produce impairment in social or occupational functioning.	63
● Are not precipitated by stress.	64
● Are prolonged (over 4 hours).	55
● Are associated with dysphoria.	65
Severe (one of the following)	
● Persistent episodes of depersonalization (24 hours and longer).	38–47, 55
● Episodes of depersonalization occur daily or weekly. May be brief or prolonged.	38–47, 54
● Frequent (more than 4) episodes of depersonalization that (one of the following)	
● Produce impairment in social or occupational functioning.	63
● Do not appear to be precipitated by stress.	64
● Are prolonged (over 4 hours).	55
● Are associated with dysphoria.	65

Note. The Severity Rating Definitions are not an inclusive list. The purpose of these definitions is to give the rater a general description of the parameters of the spectrum of dissociative symptoms and their severity.
Source. Reprinted with permission from Steinberg M: *Interviewer's Guide to the Structured Clinical Interview for DSM-IV Dissociative Disorders (SCID-D)*. Washington, DC, American Psychiatric Press, 1993. Copyright 1993 American Psychiatric Press, Inc.

"Have you ever found yourself in a place away from your home and been unable to remember who you were?" One patient described the following:

> There's just a blank there. You just have no recollection of existing at all. I can sometimes all of a sudden be in the middle of doing something, and the last memory I have was in the middle of something else totally unrelated and I could be in a different car, a different location, I could be any place that would happen. (SCID-D interview, unpublished transcript)

Question 15 asks, "Have you ever been unable to recall your name, age, address, or other important information?" Question 15 is a diagnostically discriminating question on this interview in that patients with dissociative disorders provide distinctive responses compared with nondissociative individuals. Patients with dissociative disorders who have experienced trouble remembering either their name or their age will usually answer this question by volunteering information about occasions when this occurred, as in the following example (I = interviewer; P = patient):

I: Have you ever been unable to recall your name, age, or address or other important personal information?
P: I can never remember my birthday, never.
I: So if somebody asks you when your birthday is . . . .
P: I have to struggle to remember . . . I'll find somebody who is close to my age and I'll say, "When were we born?" (SCID-D interview, unpublished interview)

Each positive response to a question on amnesia is followed up by questions designed to further explore the symptom in the patient's own words. If a patient endorses the existence of large gaps in his or her memory, follow-up questions such as "What was that experience like?" or "Can you describe what makes you aware of your memory gaps?" can help clarify the nature and extent of the amnesia.

Behavioral manifestations of amnesia that may be described during the SCID-D interview include efforts to keep track of missing time and information. For example, one patient with severe amnesia notes the number of miles on her odometer each evening and each morning in order to detect any amnesia for her use of the car during the night. Patients may also rely on other people's memories or refrain from scheduling activities because they are unable to maintain appointments.

SCID-D research indicates a spectrum of amnesia ranging from the occasional forgetfulness of normal control subjects, to the occasional or frequent memory difficulties of patients with a variety of psychiatric disorders, to recurrent or persistent episodes of amnesia (lasting days or longer) in patients with dissociative disorders. Frequent episodes of amnesia are often associated with impairment in social or occupational function, are not necessarily precipitated by external stress, are prolonged, and are usually associated with dysphoria.

Assessing depersonalization. As the following statement by Fewtrell (1986) attests, depersonalization, like amnesia, is an elusive symptom.

> [It] involves a strange absence of feeling and an apparent reduction of vividness and reality. It is therefore difficult for many people to articulate. Whereas most subjects can readily describe an anxiety bout or feelings of morbid depression, a curious state of non-being is much more difficult to put into words. (Fewtrell 1986, p. 264)

Chronic depersonalization often results in very little distress and may be seen as natural to individuals, giving them little reason to share their experience with a clinician. However, it may lead indirectly to a variety of self-destructive behaviors, the most serious of which are suicidal gestures and suicide attempts in order to regain the feeling of being alive.

The SCID-D assessment of depersonalization begins with straightforward questions that enable the patient to verbalize his or her experiences, often for the first time: question 38, "Have you ever felt that you were watching yourself from a point outside of your body, as if you were seeing yourself from a distance (or watching a movie of yourself)?"; question 40, "Have you ever had the feeling that you were a stranger to yourself?"; and question 41, "Have you ever felt as if part of your body or your whole being was foreign to you?" If the answer is "yes," the interviewer asks, "What was that experience like?" Characteristically, a patient with severe depersonalization will describe feeling as if his or her head, limbs, or entire body has become foreign or disconnected, as in the following example:

> I felt like I do not belong in this body. I, I'm in the wrong body. I don't know how to explain that . . . . I feel that I was not supposed to have been born into this body. Which body it is, I don't know. It was not this body . . . . I always felt I had the wrong face. (SCID-D interview, unpublished transcript)

Behavioral manifestations of depersonalization may include a trance-like appearance, disavowal of behaviors and talents (due to estrangement from oneself), and impaired relationships with others.

The spectrum of depersonalization has been described by numerous investigators. Normal depersonalization can be differentiated from pathological depersonalization based on the severity and context of the depersonalization symptoms. Individuals without psychiatric illness may experience episodes of depersonalization under a variety of circumstances, particularly during adolescence or as young adults (Dixon 1963; D. Myers and Grant 1972; Roberts 1960; Trueman 1984b). In college students, brief episodes of depersonalization were noted to occur in 8.5%–46% (Dixon 1963; D. Myers and Grant 1972; Trueman 1984a). Variation in the rate of depersonalization may be a function of differences in samples, questionnaires, rates of response, or methods of verifying episodes. In individuals without psychiatric illness, depersonalization may be precipitated by extreme fatigue, sensory deprivation, drug or alcohol intoxication, sleep deprivation, and severe psychosocial stress. According to Noyes and Kletti (1977), "depersonalization is, like fear, an almost universal response to life-threatening danger. It develops instantly upon the recognition of danger and vanishes just as quickly when the threat to life has passed."

On the other hand, people with dissociative disorders experience this symptom with or without prior stress, and it occurs in the absence of any single immediate psychosocial trauma (see Table 4–2 for further information). SCID-D research indicates that depersonalization in patients with dissociative disorders is accompanied by ongoing and recurrent interactive dialogues between the observing and the participating self (Steinberg 1991), as in the following example:

> I start to argue with somebody that's in that chair, but I see that person in that chair and I see it's me. I see that person and he's looking at me and he's laughing at me, and he's calling me on to fight him, and fight him, and fight him, and I don't want to fight him . . . . I see me outside myself, in other words, and he's laughing at me, calling out saying, "Come on punk, fight me, come on punk, fight me." (SCID-D interview, unpublished transcript)

In individuals without psychiatric illness, depersonalization occurs transiently and without ongoing dialogues. When dialogues occur, they retain features of memory, including memories of an actual prior conversation, or take the form of a rehearsal for an anticipated dialogue with a real person.

Table 4–2. Distinguishing between normal and pathological depersonalization

Characteristics	Common mild depersonalization	Transient depersonalization	Pathological depersonalization
Context	Occurs as an isolated symptom	Occurs as an isolated symptom	Occurs within a constellation of other dissociative or nondissociative symptoms
Frequency	One or few episodes	One episode that is transient	Persistent or recurrent depersonalization
Duration	Depersonalization episode is brief; lasts seconds to minutes	Depersonalization of limited duration (minutes to weeks)	Chronic and habitual depersonalization lasting up to many years
Precipitating factors	• Extreme fatigue • Sensory deprivation • Hypnagogic and hypnopompic states • Drug or alcohol intoxication • Sleep deprivation • Medical illness/toxic states • Severe psychosocial stress	• Life-threatening danger; this is a syndrome noted to occur in 33% of individuals immediately following exposure to life-threatening danger, such as near-death experiences and auto accidents (Noyes et al. 1977) • Single, severe psychological trauma	• Not associated with precipitating factors listed in column 1 • May be precipitated by a traumatic memory • May be precipitated by a stressful event, but occurs even when there is no stress • Occurs in the absence of a single immediate severe psychosocial trauma

Source. Reprinted with permission from Steinberg M: *Interviewer's Guide to the Structured Clinical Interview for DSM-IV Dissociative Disorders (SCID-D).* Washington, DC, American Psychiatric Press, 1993. Copyright 1993 American Psychiatric Press, Inc.

In summary, depersonalization in normal subjects differs both in nature and in persistence from that experienced by patients with psychiatric disorders. Patients with mixed psychiatric disorders also exhibit characteristic differences from those with dissociative disorders. There is a broad spectrum of depersonalization: isolated, brief episodes, usually associated with stress, in normal subjects; a few episodes to recurrent episodes in mixed psychiatric patients; and recurrent to persistent depersonalization, which may be accompanied by ongoing interactive dialogues, in patients with dissociative disorders and in PTSD (Steinberg 1991).

Assessing derealization. Derealization frequently coexists with depersonalization and only rarely occurs alone. Like depersonalization, it is often associated with a variety of perceptual distortions, including an intensification of colors, the feeling as if objects in the environment are changing in size, and a general sense of estrangement from one's surroundings. Derealization commonly involves the feeling that friends or relatives have lost their normal sense of familiarity.

SCID-D questions on derealization include question 79, "Have you ever felt as if familiar surroundings or people you knew seemed unfamiliar or unreal?," and question 84, "Have you ever felt puzzled as to what is real and what is unreal in your surroundings?" Patients with severe derealization describe recurrent feelings that close relatives, particularly their parents, are unreal and that their own home is foreign to them. Often, these feelings are associated with traumatic memories of childhood events that patients may spontaneously share when describing intense derealization experiences. When asked about derealization, patients with severe dissociative symptomatology may also describe flashbacks and age regressed states that were accompanied by derealization (Boon and Draijer 1991).

In derealization, the individual often experiences incongruent feelings or perceptions about familiar people:

> I would think to myself, "Who is this person, it isn't my mother." I would hear myself thinking, "This person isn't my mother. Who is this person? She's not my mother." (SCID-D interview, unpublished transcript)

Such experiences should be distinguished from amnestic episodes in which the patient would be asking simply "Who is this person?" There would be an inability to recognize the identity of the person near her rather than a feeling that "this is not my mother."

Behavioral manifestations of derealization may include failure to interact appropriately with relatives and/or close friends and attempts to orient oneself in one's environment by identifying personal belongings.

The spectrum of derealization ranges from isolated, brief episodes associated with stress, fatigue, drugs, or alcohol in normal subjects and isolated to recurrent derealization episodes in mixed psychiatric patients, to recurrent derealization in patients with PTSD and the dissociative disorders.

Assessing identity confusion.   The SCID-D interview may elicit a variety of thematic clues that suggest the presence of identity confusion, including the theme of an inner battle regarding one's identity.

Questions about identity confusion include question 102, "Have you ever felt as if there was a struggle going on inside of you about who you really are?," and question 105, "Have you ever felt confused as to who you are?" People with severe dissociative symptoms will often answer these questions with "all the time." In the following excerpt from an unpublished SCID-D interview, the patient describes how vividly this internal struggle manifests itself.

> **I:** Have you ever felt as if there is a struggle going on inside of you?
>
> **P:** Yes.
>
> **I:** What's that like?
>
> **P:** I just told you about it, that person that wants to come out. He struggles, struggles with me. And this guy must think I'm nuts, if I'm gonna let him out. If I let him out, I'm never gonna get myself back in. And that's what scares me the most.
>
> **I:** What's the struggle like?
>
> **P:** It's like a tug of war. Pulling, pulling the rope, pulling, you keep pulling and pulling, and he pulls you back and you pull it forward, and he pulls you back, and you pull it forward, and you want to say, "Hey, man. Take the damn thing." You know. And I keep pulling that rope, and he keeps pulling it back, and I pull it again. (Raises voice and sounds very aggravated.) One of these days, he might win. (SCID-D interview, unpublished transcript)

As with the other dissociative symptoms, there is a spectrum of identity confusion. In normal adults, questions about identity confusion are answered either negatively or are answered in terms of an effort to integrate one's various roles (e.g., daughter, wife, mother, professional). Such a response would be rated as "mild." In patients with mixed psychiatric disorders, including schizophrenia, identity confusion is described in terms of a struggle to find an appropriate role in the world. On the other hand, patients with severe dissociative pathology describe a persistent internal struggle/uncertainty as to their identity. This is usually associated with distress and/or dysfunction.

Assessing identity alteration.   Often, the subjective sense of identity confusion will have behavioral manifestations of which the patient may or may not be fully aware. For the purposes of the SCID-D, such external manifestations of identity confusion are categorized as identity alteration. Some questions about identity alteration include question 116, "Have you ever been told by others that you seem like a different person?," and question 118, "Have you ever referred to yourself (or been told by others that you referred to yourself) by different names (other than nicknames or name changes due to marriage)?"

Patients with dissociative disorders often report that they have found themselves using different names or acting like a different person. They may also report that others have frequently brought such behavior to their attention, though they themselves have amnesia for their identity alteration. Other examples of identity alteration include third-person references to the self, use of different names, and alterations in skills or capabilities without apparent reason. The concealment of awareness of these symptoms of identity alteration may be due to amnesia or avoidance:

> **I:**   You mentioned that people have told you you have used different names. You mentioned Jennifer and Mary. What other names have they mentioned?
>
> **P:**   Sue, Tracy, Donna. I don't know that I can recite them accurately.
>
> **I:**   What do they say about Sue or Tracy or Donna?
>
> **P:**   Sue is vicious and Tracy is mean. This sounds really stupid. Frank, my friend, told me, "Just let me know when Sue arrives. She has a black belt in karate and I don't want to deal with it." I mean, how can your friend tell you that you have a black belt, and I don't even know karate. I'm not very athletic either. Ahh, I don't know . . . the only thing that bothers me is the consis-

tency of them between different people; they're still close
enough to raise questions, you know what I mean? They're not
sporadic. They're very close to each other, even though they
don't know each other.

I: So how do you understand it?

P: Well, I always look at it like a fluke of nature and I just prefer
not to deal with it. (SCID-D interview, unpublished transcript)

Responses to SCID-D questions have represented a spectrum of identity
alteration. Subjects without psychiatric disorders will either report no history or describe mild identity alteration in which they assume different roles
or demeanors but are aware of these roles or feel that they are in their
control. This is generally not associated with dysfunction or dysphoria. Patients with mixed psychiatric disorders (such as manic depressive illness)
may report alterations in behavior/demeanor that are not in their control.
However, these alterations do not appear to represent distinct personalities.
Patients with DID have experienced alterations in their identity representing
distinct personalities that appear to take control of their behavior, speech,
demeanor, and so on. Patients with PTSD often describe symptoms of identity confusion and alteration reflecting a shift in their behavior and/or identity from the current characteristics of their personality to those operative at
the time they experienced the trauma.

ASSESSING THE DISSOCIATIVE
DISORDERS AND PTSD

Dissociative Disorders

The five dissociative disorders in DSM-IV, dissociative amnesia, dissociative
fugue, depersonalization disorder, DID, and DDNOS, can be assessed in
terms of constellations of the five dissociative symptoms discussed in the
previous section. Based on SCID-D research, there are specific symptom
profiles for the dissociative disorders (see Figure 4–1; Steinberg 1993b;
Steinberg et al. 1990; Steinberg 1989–1992).

Dissociative amnesia. The DSM-IV diagnostic criteria for dissociative
amnesia are the following:

- The predominant disturbance is one or more episodes of inability to recall important personal information, usually of a traumatic or stressful nature, that is too extensive to be explained by ordinary forgetfulness.
- The disturbance does not occur exclusively during the course of DID, dissociative fugue, PTSD, acute stress disorder, or somatization disorder and is not due to the direct physiological effects of a substance (e.g., a drug of abuse, medication) or a neurological or other general medical condition (e.g., amnestic disorder due to head trauma).
- The symptoms cause clinically significant distress or impairment in social, occupational, or other important areas of functioning. (p. 481)

Therefore, dissociative amnesia consists of the psychogenic symptom of amnesia, in the absence of significant depersonalization, derealization, identity confusion, and identity alteration associated with other dissociative, traumatic stress-related, or somatization disorders. If any of the other four dissociative symptoms are present to a significant degree, the diagnosis of dissociative amnesia is ruled out.

There are distinguishing features of the amnesia present in patients with dissociative amnesia. The onset is usually abrupt and follows severe stress. Termination of the amnesia also tends to be abrupt, with complete recovery and rare recurrences. If a patient experiences *recurrent* amnestic episodes, one should rule out the presence of another dissociative disorder such as DID and DDNOS.

Dissociative fugue. The DSM-IV criteria for dissociative fugue are the following:

- The predominant disturbance is sudden, unexpected travel away from home or one's customary place of work, with inability to recall one's past.
- Confusion about personal identity or assumption of new identity (partial or complete).
- The disturbance does not occur exclusively during the course of DID and is not due to the direct physiological effects of a substance (e.g., a drug of abuse, medication) or a general medical condition (e.g., temporal lobe epilepsy).
- The symptoms cause clinically significant distress or impairment in social, occupational, or other important areas of functioning. (p. 484)

Fugue states therefore consist of the symptom of amnesia in severe form, along with identity confusion and/or alteration. There may also be amnesia for the episode after the patient has emerged from the fugue state, perhaps as a result of state-dependent encoding of memory (Kihlstrom 1993).

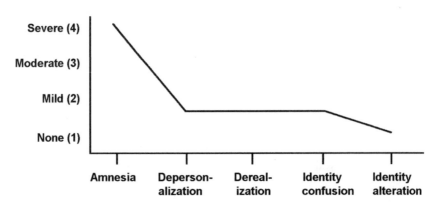

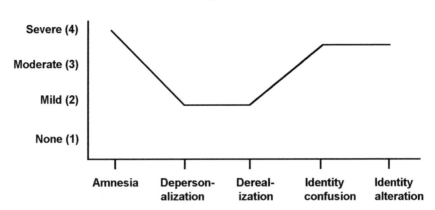

Figure 4–1. Symptom profiles of the dissociative disorders.
Source. Reprinted with permission from Steinberg M: *Interviewer's Guide to the Structured Clinical Interview for DSM-IV Dissociative Disorders (SCID-D).* Washington, DC, American Psychiatric Press, 1993. Copyright 1993 American Psychiatric Press, Inc.

As with dissociative amnesia, DID and organic disorders must be ruled out to justify a diagnosis of dissociative fugue. Episodes of fugue are usually brief and rarely reoccur.

Depersonalization disorder. Depersonalization disorder consists of persistent or recurrent experiences of depersonalization that cause marked distress or dysfunction. Patients with depersonalization may experience derealization and identity confusion, solely in conjunction with their deper-

Depersonalization disorder

Dissociative identity disorder (DID) and Dissociative disorder not otherwise specified (DDNOS)

Figure 4–1. Symptom profiles of the dissociative disorders (continued).

sonalization. Significant derealization or identity confusion occurring independently from the depersonalization would rule out depersonalization disorder. Similarly, significant identity alteration would suggest the presence of another dissociative disorder such as DID or DDNOS. The existence of schizophrenia, substance use, or a medical condition as a precipitating factor would also rule out depersonalization disorder.

DID. DSM-IV criteria for DID are the following:

- The presence of two or more distinct identities or personality states (each with its own relatively enduring pattern of perceiving, relating to, and thinking about the environment and self).
- At least two of these identities or personality states recurrently take control of the person's behavior.
- Inability to recall important personal information that is too extensive to be explained by ordinary forgetfulness.
- The disturbance is not due to the direct physiological effects of a substance (e.g., blackouts or chaotic behavior during alcohol intoxication) or a general medical condition (e.g., complex partial seizures). (p. 487)

Exclusionary factors include substance use and medical condition. Therefore, by use of these criteria, the predominant underlying symptoms of DID are manifestations of severe amnesia and severe identity alteration. Most patients with DID also experience severe depersonalization, derealization, and identity confusion. However, as a result of the amnesia, the patient may deny experiencing these symptoms.

To overcome the amnestic barrier, the SCID-D supplements questions investigating the patient's subjective awareness with questions referring to the reports of other observers. For example, question 114, "Have you ever acted as if you were a completely different person?," is followed by question 116, "Have you ever been told by others that you seem like a different person?"

The follow-up sections of the SCID-D (questions 159–258) enable the interviewer to assess the extent of a patient's identity alteration in order to consider the presence of two or more personalities. The interview explores whether dissociative experiences control the patient's behavior or speech; whether there is a particular name, age, visual appearance, demeanor, behavioral pattern, or life history associated with the symptoms the patient has acknowledged; and whether these symptoms reflect distinct identities or personality states. For example, the follow-up section on "different person" seeks to clarify and expand on earlier responses indicating that the patient has felt/acted like a different person. As in all sections of the SCID-D, each affirmative response is followed by a request for descriptive elaboration such as "Can you say anything more about that?" or "What is that experience like?"

Patients with DID often describe vividly the existence of two or more people who control their emotions, speech, and behavior. An associated feature of the identity confusion and identity alteration associated with DID is the feeling that different parts of one's brain contain different personality states and/or personalities. Patients may report an internal architecture inhabited by alternate personalities, as in the following example:

> All of the parts inside of me have rooms. Every room is different. My room is at the far end and there's more space between my door and the door next to me. Diana's room has walls made out of mahogany. She has three big huge windows and she looks out onto a garden. Um. Julia's room has bunk beds in it and a rug on the floor and teddy bears and dolls and stuff like that in it. Every room is different. (SCID-D interview, unpublished transcript)

DDNOS. DDNOS is a category for dissociative disorders in which the predominant feature is a dissociative symptom or syndrome (i.e., a disruption in the usually integrated functions of consciousness, identity, memory, or perception of the environment) that does not meet the criteria for any of the specific dissociative disorders in DSM-IV. Various constellations of the five dissociative symptoms may qualify for the diagnosis of DDNOS. Diagnoses include cases similar to DID but lacking sufficiently distinct personalities or amnesia for important personal information, the experience of derealization unaccompanied by depersonalization, coercive persuasion in hostages or cult victims, and trance states leading to distress or impairment.

Diagnostic categories for DSM-IV. Diagnostic assessments obtained with the SCID-D are consistent with the criteria adopted in DSM-IV. New categories in the dissociative disorders can also be assessed with the SCID-D. *Dissociative trance disorder* includes "culturally patterned dissociative syndromes" (D. Spiegel and Cardeña 1991, p. 375) such as "involuntary possession states" and other dissociative phenomena that result in distress and dysfunction. In dissociative trance disorder, the trance or possession state is not accepted as a normal part of a collective cultural or religious practice and is not due to DID, a psychotic disorder, substance use, or a medical condition.

Cross-cultural descriptions of possession and trance-like states suggest the presence of the five dissociative symptoms. Individuals undergoing possession or trance often experience amnesia associated with these episodes, experience a sense of estrangement from themselves and their environment (depersonalization and derealization), and exhibit identity alteration, with such behavioral manifestations as speaking in a different voice and assuming an alternate identity (Cardeña 1991; Jenson, in press; Saxena and Presad 1989).

The new criteria for *acute stress disorder (acute anxiety and dissociative disorder)* include exposure to a traumatic event that is associated with the development of dissociative symptoms, including depersonalization, derealization, and amnesia, as well as anxiety symptoms. In order to receive a diagnosis of acute stress disorder (acute anxiety and dissociative disorder), the symptoms must cause significant impairment or distress but must last less than 4 weeks.

PTSD

Given the posttraumatic etiology of the dissociative disorders (Coons et al. 1989; Kluft 1988, 1991; D. Spiegel 1984; Spiegel and Cardeña 1991), it is not surprising that patients with PTSD also suffer severe dissociative symptoms, including "radical discontinuities in their conscious memories of trauma in such a manner that these memories are kept separate from other memories or components of the patient's identity" (Spiegel and Cardeña 1991, p. 29). Dissociative symptoms such as depersonalization, derealization, and amnesia are prominent components of PTSD (Spiegel and Cardeña 1991) and can be systematically assessed using the SCID-D interview.

Patients with PTSD may describe episodes in which their behavior/identity shifts between that of an individual living in the present and that of a younger individual (their past self) who is experiencing immediate trauma. Such episodes of age regression and flashbacks (phenomena commonly associated with PTSD and the dissociative disorders) may also be conceptualized in terms of the five core dissociative symptoms (Steinberg 1989–1992). Age regression, "reliving the past as though it were occurring in the present, with age appropriate vocabulary, mental content, and affect" (D. Spiegel and Rosenfeld 1984, p. 522), involves identity alteration and derealization. Variable amounts of amnesia, depersonalization, and identity confusion may also be present. Patients experiencing flashbacks may experience depersonalization and derealization during these episodes and may be amnestic for the flashbacks.

CONCLUSION

Although dissociation is a complex and multifaceted phenomenon, the varied presentations of dissociation need not impede diagnostic accuracy. I have suggested a model on the basis of which dissociation can be organized and systematically assessed. A growing body of SCID-D research indicates striking consistency in the clinical phenomenology of dissociation with respect to five dissociative symptoms (i.e., amnesia, depersonalization, derealization, identity confusion, and identity alteration) and several disorders (Boon and Draijer 1991; Goff et al. 1992; Steinberg 1993a, 1993b; Steinberg 1989–1992; Steinberg et al. 1990; Steinberg et al. 1989–1993). The dissociative symptoms of patients with dissociative disorders and PTSD differ both qualitatively and quantitatively from those experienced by patients with other psychiatric disorders and from the transient episodes that can occur in normal subjects. Virtually identical results have been obtained at multiple sites using the SCID-D. Continued experimental and clinical research with the SCID-D will provide a more detailed understanding of dissociative phenomena.

REFERENCES

Ackner B: Depersonalization; I: aetiology and phenomenology. Journal of Mental Science 100:838–853, 1954

Akhtar S, Brenner I: Differential diagnosis of fugue-like states. J Clin Psychiatry 40:381–385, 1979

American Psychiatric Association: Diagnostic and Statistical Manual of Mental Disorders, 4th Edition. Washington, DC, American Psychiatric Association, 1994

Bernstein E, Putnam FW: Development, reliability, and validity of a dissociation scale. J Nerv Ment Dis 174:727–735, 1986

Bliss E, Jeppsen E: Prevalence of multiple personality among inpatients and outpatients. Am J Psychiatry 142:250–251, 1985

Boon S, Draijer N: Diagnosing dissociative disorders in the Netherlands: a pilot study with the Structured Clinical Interview for DSM-III-R Dissociative Disorders. Am J Psychiatry 148:458–462, 1991

Bowers K: Unconscious influence and hypnosis, in Repression and Dissociation: Implications for Personality Theory, Psychopathology, and Health. Edited by Singer JL. Chicago, IL, University of Chicago Press, 1990, pp 143–179

Brauer R, Harrow M, Tucker G: Depersonalization phenomena in psychiatric patients. Br J Psychiatry 117:509–515, 1970

Braun B: Towards a theory of multiple personality and other dissociative phenomena, in Symposium on Multiple Personality. Edited by Braun BG. Psychiatr Clin North Am 7:171–193, 1984

Briere J, Conte J: Amnesia in adults molested as children: testing theories of repression. Paper presented at the 97th Annual Convention of the American Psychological Association, New Orleans, LA, August, 11–15 1989

Bryer J, Nelson B, Miller J, et al: Childhood sexual and physical abuse as factors in adult psychiatric illness. Am J Psychiatry 144:1426–1430, 1987

Cardeña E: The varieties of possession experience. Association for the Anthropological Study of Consciousness Quarterly 5:1–17, 1991

Cattell J: Depersonalization: psychological and social perspectives, in American Handbook of Psychiatry, 2nd Edition. Edited by Arieti S. New York, Basic Books, 1975, pp 766–799

Cicchetti DV, Sparrow S: Developing criteria for establishing interrater reliability of specific items: applications to assessment of adaptive behavior. American Journal of Mental Deficiency 86:127–137, 1981

Coons PM: The differential diagnosis of multiple personality: a comprehensive review. Psychiatr Clin North Am 12:51–67, 1984

Coons P, Bowman E, Milstein V: Multiple personality disorder: a clinical investigation of 50 cases. J Nerv Ment Dis 176:519–527, 1988

Coons P, Bowman E, Pellow TA: Post-traumatic aspects of the treatment of victims of sexual abuse and incest. Psychiatr Clin North Am 12:325–337, 1989

Davison K: Episodic depersonalization: observations on 7 patients. Br J Psychiatry 110:505–513, 1964

Dixon J: Depersonalization phenomena in a sample population of college students. Br J Psychiatry 109:371–375, 1963

Edwards G, Angus J: Depersonalization. Br J Psychiatry 120:242–244, 1972

Ellenberger H: The Discovery of the Unconscious: The History and Evolution of Dynamic Psychiatry. New York, Basic Books, 1970

Ellerstein N, Canavan J: Sexual abuse of boys. Am J Dis Child 134:250–257, 1980

Emslie G, Rosenfelt A: Incest reported by children and adolescents hospitalized for severe psychiatric problems. Am J Psychiatry 140:708–711, 1983

Erdelyi M: Psychoanalysis: Freud's Cognitive Psychology. New York, Freeman, 1985

Fewtrell W: Depersonalization: a description and suggested strategies. British Journal of Guidance and Counseling 14:263–269, 1986

Fine C: The cognitive sequelae of incest, in Incest-Related Syndromes of Adult Psychopathology. Edited by Kluft R. Washington, DC, American Psychiatric Press, 1990, pp 161–182

Fink D, Golinkoff M: Multiple personality disorder, borderline personality disorder and schizophrenia: a comparative study of clinical features. Dissociation 3:127–134, 1990

Fleiss J: Statistical Methods for Rates and Proportions. New York, Wiley, 1981

Frankel F: Hypnotizability and dissociation. Am J Psychiatry 147:823–829, 1990

Freud S: The Unconscious (1915), in The Standard Edition of the Complete Psychological Works of Sigmund Freud, Vol 14. Translated and edited by Strachey J. London, Hogarth Press, 1963, pp 159–215

Frischholz E: The relationship among dissociation, hypnosis, and child abuse in the development of multiple personality disorder, in Childhood Antecedents of Multiple Personality. Edited by Kluft RP. Washington, DC, American Psychiatric Press, 1985, pp 99–126

Galdston I: On the etiology of depersonalization. J Nerv Ment Dis 105:25–39, 1947

Goff DC, Olin JA, Jenike MA, et al: Dissociative symptoms in patients with obsessive-compulsive disorder. J Nerv Ment Dis 180:332–337, 1992

Goodwin J: Credibility problems in multiple personality disorder patients and abused children, in Childhood Antecedents of Multiple Personality. Edited by Kluft RP. Washington, DC, American Psychiatric Press, 1985, pp 1–19

Goodwin J: Posttraumatic symptoms in abused children. Journal of Traumatic Stress 1:475–488, 1988

Hart B: The conception of the subconsciousness. J Abnorm Psychol 4:351–371, 1910

Hart B: The conception of dissociation. Br J Med Psychol 6:241–263, 1926

Hilgard ER: Divided Consciousness: Multiple Controls in Human Thought and Action, Expanded Edition. New York, Wiley, 1986

Horevitz R, Braun B: Are multiple personalities borderline? Psychiatr Clin North Am 7:69–87, 1984

Husain A, Chapel J: History of incest in girls admitted to a psychiatric hospital. Am J Psychiatry 140:591–593, 1983

Jenson G: Conclusions and implications of trance and possession for multiple personality, suicide, and mental health, in Trance and Possession in Bali: A Window on Multiple Personality and Suicide. Edited by Suryani L, Jenson G. Singapore, Oxford University Press (in press)

Kiersch T: Amnesia: a clinical study of ninety-eight cases. Am J Psychiatry 119:57–60, 1962

Kihlstrom J: The cognitive unconscious. Science 237:1445–1452, 1987

Kihlstrom J, Hoyt I: Repression, dissociation, and hypnosis, in Repression and Dissociation. Edited by Singer J. Chicago, IL, University of Chicago Press, 1990, pp 181–208

Kihlstrom J: Dissociative Disorders, in Comprehensive Handbook of Psychopathology, 2nd Edition. Edited by Sutker P, Adams H. New York, Plenum, 1993

Kirshner L: Dissociative reactions: an historical review and clinical study. Acta Psychiatr Scand 49:698–711, 1973

Kluft R: Aspects of the treatment of multiple personality disorder. Psychiatric Annals 14:51–55, 1984a

Kluft R: Treatment of multiple personality: a study of 33 cases. Psychiatr Clin North Am 7:9–29, 1984b

Kluft R: The natural history of multiple personality disorder, in Childhood Antecedents of Multiple Personality. Edited by Kluft R. Washington, DC, American Psychiatric Press, 1985, pp 197–238

Kluft R: The dissociative disorders, in The American Psychiatric Press Textbook of Psychiatry. Edited by Talbott J, Hales R, Yudofsky S. Washington, DC, American Psychiatric Press, 1988, pp 557–585

Kluft RP: Multiple personality disorder, in American Psychiatric Press Review of Psychiatry, Vol 10. Edited by Tasman A, Goldfinger SM. Washington, DC, American Psychiatric Association Press, 1991, pp 161–188

Levy J, Wachtel P: Depersonalization: an effort at clarification. Am J Psychoanal 38:291–300, 1978

Loewenstein RJ: Psychogenic amnesia and psychogenic fugue: a comprehensive review, in American Psychiatric Press Review of Psychiatry, Vol 10. Edited by Tasman A, Goldfinger SM. Washington, DC, American Psychiatric Association Press, 1991, pp 189–222

Mayer-Gross W: On depersonalization. Br J Med Psychol 15:103–126, 1935

Münsterberg H: A symposium of the subconscious. J Abnorm Psychol 2:25–33, 1907

Myers F: Human Personality and Its Survival of Bodily Death. Vols 1 & 2. London, Longmans, Green, & Company, 1903

Myers M: Physical and sexual abuse histories of male psychiatric patients (letter). Am J Psychiatry 148:399, 1991

Myers D, Grant G: A study of depersonalization in students. Br J Psychiatry 121:59–65, 1972

Nemiah J: Dissociative disorders, in Comprehensive Textbook of Psychiatry, 4th Edition. Edited by Kaplan H, Sadock B. Baltimore, MD, Williams & Wilkins, 1985, pp 942–957

Nemiah JC: Dissociation, conversion, and somatization, in American Psychiatric Press Review of Psychiatry, Vol 10. Edited by Tasman A, Goldfinger SM. Washington, DC, American Psychiatric Press, 1991, pp 248–260

Noyes R Jr, Kletti R: Depersonalization in response to life-threatening danger. Compr Psychiatry 18:375–384, 1977

Prince M: A symposium on the subconscious. J Abnorm Psychol 2:67–80, 1907

Putnam F, Guroff J, Silberman E, et al: The clinical phenomenology of multiple personality disorder: review of 100 recent cases. J Clin Psychiatry 47:285–293, 1986

Quen J (ed): Split Minds Split Brains: Historical and Current Perspectives. New York, New York University Press, 1986

Reed GF: The Psychology of Anomalous Experience. Buffalo, NY, Prometheus Books, 1988

Riley K: Measurement of dissociation. J Nerv Ment Dis 176:449–450, 1988

Roberts W: Normal and abnormal depersonalization. Journal of Mental Science 106:478–493, 1960

Rosenfeld A: Incidence of history of incest among 18 female psychiatric patients. Am J Psychiatry 136:791–795, 1979

Ross C, Norton G: Multiple personality disorder patients with a prior diagnosis of schizophrenia. Dissociation 1:39–42, 1988

Ross CA, Heber S, Norton GR, et al: The Dissociative Disorders Interview Schedule: a structured interview. Dissociation 2,3:169–189, 1989

Sansonnet-Hayden H, Haley G, Marriage K, et al: Sexual abuse and psychopathology in hospitalized adolescents. J Am Acad Child Adolescent Psychiatry 26:753–757, 1987

Saperstein J: On the phenomenon of depersonalization. J Nerv Ment Dis 110:236–251, 1949

Sanders S: The perceptual alteration scale: a scale measuring dissociation. Am J Clin Hypn 29:95–102, 1986

Saxena S, Prasad K: DSM-III subclassification of dissociative disorders applied to psychiatric outpatients in India. Am J Psychiatry 146:261–262, 1989

Schacter D, Kihlstrom J: Functional amnesia, in Handbook of Neuropsychology. Edited by Boller F, Grafman J. New York, Elsevier Science Publishers, 1989, pp 209–231

Schultz R, Braun B, Kluft R: Multiple personality disorder: phenomenology of selected variables in comparison to major depression. Dissociation 2:45–51, 1989

Sidis B: The Psychology of Suggestion. New York, Appleton, 1911

Singer J, Sincoff J: Summary: beyond repression and the defenses, in Repression and Dissociation. Edited by Singer J. Chicago, IL, University of Chicago Press, 1990, pp 471–496

Siomopoulos V: Derealization and déjà vu: formal mechanisms. Am J Psychotherapy 26:84–89, 1972

Spiegel D: Multiple personality as a post-traumatic stress disorder. Psychiatr Clin North Am 7:101–110, 1984

Spiegel D: Hypnosis, dissociation and trauma: hidden and overt observers, in Repression and Dissociation. Edited by Singer J. Chicago, IL, University of Chicago Press, 1990, pp 121–142

Spiegel D: Dissociation and trauma, in American Psychiatric Press Review of Psychiatry, Vol 10. Edited by Tasman A, Goldfinger SM. Washington, DC, American Psychiatric Association Press, 1991, pp 261–275

Spiegel D, Cardeña E: Disintegrated experience: the dissociative disorders revisited. J Abnorm Psychol 100:366–378, 1991

Spiegel D, Rosenfeld A: Spontaneous hypnotic age regression: case report. J Clin Psychiatry 45:522–524, 1984

Spiegel H, Spiegel D: Trance and Treatment: Clinical Uses of Hypnosis. Washington, DC, American Psychiatric Press, 1987

Spitzer R, Williams J, Gibbon M, et al: Structured Clinical Interview for DSM-III-R (SCID). Washington, DC, American Psychiatric Press, 1990

Steinberg M: Structured Clinical Interview for DSM-III-R Dissociative Disorders (SCID-D). New Haven, CT, Yale University School of Medicine, 1985

Steinberg M (Principal Investigator): NIMH-Funded Field Trials of the Structured Clinical Interview for DSM-III-R Dissociative Disorders (SCID-D). New Haven, CT, Yale University School of Medicine, 1989–1992

Steinberg M: The Spectrum of depersonalization: assessment and treatment, in American Psychiatric Press Review of Psychiatry, Vol 10. Edited by Tasman A, Goldfinger SM. Washington, DC, American Psychiatric Press, 1991, pp 223–247

Steinberg M: Structured Clinical Interview for DSM-IV Dissociative Disorders (SCID-D). Washington, DC, American Psychiatric Press, 1993a

Steinberg M: Interviewer's Guide to the Structured Clinical Interview for DSM-IV Dissociative Disorders (SCID-D). Washington, DC, American Psychiatric Press, 1993b

Steinberg M, Howland F, Cicchetti DV: The Structured Clinical Interview for DSM-III-R Dissociative Disorders, in Proceedings of the International Conference on Multiple Personality and Dissociative States. Edited by Braun B. Chicago, IL, Rush Presbyterian Hospital, 1986

Steinberg M, Rounsaville BJ, Cicchetti DV: The Structured Clinical Interview for DSM-III-R Dissociative Disorders: preliminary report on a new diagnostic instrument. Am J Psychiatry 147:76–82, 1990

Steinberg M, Kluft RP, Coons PM, et al: Multicenter Field Trials of the Structured Clinical Interview for DSM-IV Dissociative Disorders (SCID-D). New Haven, CT, Yale University School of Medicine, 1989–1993

Terr L: Childhood traumas: an outline and overview. Am J Psychiatry 148:10–20, 1991

Trueman D: Anxiety and depersonalization and derealization experiences. Psychol Rep 54:91–96, 1984a

Trueman D: Depersonalization in a non-clinical population. J Psychol 116:107–112, 1984b

Section III

Culture and Dissociation

CHAPTER 5

Pacing the Void: Social and Cultural Dimensions of Dissociation

Laurence J. Kirmayer, M.D., F.R.C.P.C.

A young Tamil woman in Malaysia stands quietly amid a circle of devotees, eyes closed, face smooth, slowly swaying. Under the guidance of her guru, she has worked many evenings to prepare for this ritual. Now her guru rubs holy ash on her cheeks and pierces them clear through with a long steel spike. She does not flinch—just continues to sway, adorned with the awkward spike, oblivious to this world.

An American veteran of Vietnam, dressed in hospital gown, grips the arms of his chair, wide-eyed with emotion. Under the guidance of his psychotherapist, through hypnosis, he uncovers the memory of the death of his adopted Vietnamese son in an accidental bombing run. He shouts in fear and cries torrents of grief as he relives the events as though they are unfolding before him this instant.

A woman talks of people who live within her, sharing her body and wrestling for control of her mind. She knows of their presence by telltale traces: gaps in her memory, unaccounted mileage on her car, injuries she

This chapter was based on a presentation to the MacArthur Foundation Mind-Body Network Workshop on Dissociation, Stanford, California, October 17, 1991. I thank Joel Paris, Raymond Prince, and David Spiegel for their helpful comments on an earlier version of this chapter.

does not recall receiving. After psychotherapy with hypnosis to bridge her many selves, she remembers fleeing to a motel, slashing herself with a knife in rage, and then feeling only relief and detachment. She is now sickened to think of her self-mutilation.

These accounts mark off the domain of *dissociation* (Putnam 1991).[1] Each involves striking gaps in awareness, memory, or identity. *Dissociation* is a term applied both to the experience or behavioral expression of the gap and to the underlying mechanisms posited to account for such disruptions in the normal integration of memory, identity, and experience (E. R. Hilgard 1977; Spiegel and Cardeña 1991).

Although the drama of these examples commands attention, it may also impede our understanding of dissociation. Such arresting vignettes make dissociative phenomena like ecstatic or possession trance, clinical hypnosis, functional amnesias, and multiple personality appear to be extraordinary events, quite unrelated to ordinary psychology. Further, the very unfamiliarity of these events may blind us to their diversity, and so, lumping them all together, we may assume a priori that there is a single unique state or process that characterizes dissociation. This is the fallacy of essentialism—that is, the unwarranted assumption that an underlying essence characterizes a complex family of phenomena.

Yet, if *dissociation* names a domain of diverse phenomena related by family resemblance, they may have no single essence to be discovered by psychometrics or neurophysiology. If dissociative phenomena do have an obvious common feature, it is a negative one: They are ruptures in the normally expected integration of psychological functions and the social presentation of the self. Because there are many types of integration of different functions, it follows that there are many forms of dissociation. Similarly, there are multiple mechanisms that could interact to give rise to each form of dissociative experience. These mechanisms include cognitive, emotional, and social processes occurring at different levels of organization. Consequently, there may be no simple isomorphism between the phenomena of dissociation and underlying neurophysiological mechanisms.

In this chapter then, I will argue that dissociative phenomena—like those of hypnosis—are heterogeneous and may involve several distinct pat-

---

[1] Each of these vignettes is based on a film or videotape presented at the MacArthur Foundation Mind-Body Network Workshop on Dissociation, Stanford, California, October 16, 1991.

terns of interaction of psychological processes. Although this diversity of forms of dissociation does not invalidate the existence of a category of dissociative disorders, or the search for common features among these disorders, it does present an obstacle for research that aims to identify a single dissociative *state* or process to measure its physiological or clinical correlates. Dissociation involves multiple components or dimensions that are tapped by different measures. Decomposition of the concept of dissociation can therefore contribute to the ability to identify homogeneous groups or discrete processes in research.

The long-standing controversy in the literature of hypnosis between *state* and *social-psychological* theorists is pertinent to current models of dissociation. State or special-process theorists have argued that distinctive cognitive mechanisms underlie hypnosis (e.g., E. R. Hilgard 1977; Bowers 1991), whereas social-psychological theorists (e.g., Sarbin 1989; Spanos 1986) insist that there is no evidence for a distinctive hypnotic state or process and view hypnotic behavior and experience as the result of strategic social enactment akin to role playing. The labels are those applied by social-psychological theorists to their opponents and themselves and are misleading in that state theorists do not deny the role of social factors (e.g., E. R. Hilgard 1977; Orne 1962), and social-psychological theorists usually offer a very limited account of social processes. Both positions have had heuristic value in leading researchers to identify individual trait and social-contextual variables that influence hypnotic phenomena. Most current researchers would resist being confined to one theoretical camp, and the most interesting contemporary accounts attempt to integrate these perspectives by studying the interaction of individual traits, instructional sets, and social contexts on hypnosis (e.g., Nadon et al. 1991). The resulting interactive models allow a place for various forms of dissociation in hypnosis. I will borrow heavily from such integrative perspectives to outline the role of social factors in clinical dissociative phenomena.

In the first section, I briefly review what is known about components of dissociation and hypnosis. The second section considers the range of processes that may contribute to dissociative phenomena. The third section leads us from the interaction of mental mechanisms outward to an emphasis on the social shaping of dissociation. Because clinical and laboratory studies of dissociative disorders and hypnosis usually ignore their own social and historical context, they cannot reveal how dissociative phenomena are the outcome of beliefs and practices that differ substantially across cultures and historical periods. The final section considers the role of social and cultural factors in the integration of the personality and the production of dissociative identity disorder (DID; formerly called multiple personality disorder).

VARIETIES OF DISSOCIATIVE EXPERIENCE

The Thaipusam festival depicted in the film *Floating on Air, Followed by the Wind* (Simons and Pfaff 1973)—from which the opening example of the Tamil woman is sketched—illustrates how difficult it is to sort out fact from artifact in this area. The ritual is colorful and exotic, taking place each year in the Batu caves outside of Kuala Lumpur. We are impressed by the celebrants' lack of pain as they are pierced repeatedly with decorative skewers and hooks and their endurance as they carry heavy flower-bedecked cages to fulfill their promise to the god Murugan. There is an awesome sense that some obscure power is being revealed.

Taken as a whole, the Thaipusam ritual is extraordinarily complex and orchestrates several different processes that contribute to the celebrants' control of pain and physical endurance (Simons et al. 1988). Practice with others in the days preceding the festival gives models for trance behavior. Indeed, many participants have observed the proceedings since childhood. Participants learn to focus their attention and become absorbed in their own bodily feelings and imaginings. They may acquire conditioned cues to narrow and shift their attention inward. During practice sessions, the group provides social support and ratification for appropriate trance experience and behavior. Participants then have high expectations and much pressure to perform well before others during the festival. They expect that they will be possessed by the god Murugan who will protect them from pain.

This expectation points to one basic mechanism for pain control distinct from dissociation as such. As is well known from studies of placebo, the expectation of pain relief alone can lead to substantial analgesia (Evans 1985). The analgesic placebo effect is blocked by the opioid antagonist naloxone, suggesting that it is mediated by endorphins (Levine et al. 1978). Thus the symbolic stimuli of the ritual and the participants' expectation of pain relief from the god's intercession can evoke pain control independent of any indication of the absorption of trance or dissociation. As well, pain and stress themselves can trigger endorphin release with subsequent analgesia (Willer et al. 1981) or emotional *numbing* (Glover 1992). The intense emotion that may be associated with this important religious event may further activate endogenous pain control systems.

This is not the whole story, though, for it is likely that participants use other mechanisms of pain control that fall within the domain of dissociation. Indeed, hypnotically susceptible subjects can achieve higher levels of pain control with hypnosis than with placebo alone (McGlashan et al. 1969). There is good evidence from several studies that hypnotic analgesia is not blocked by naloxone and hence is not primarily mediated by endorphin pathways (Barber and Mayer 1977). Instead, hypnosis appears to involve higher level changes in perception and in the cognitive-emotional evaluation of and response to pain stimuli (Chaves 1989; E. R. Hilgard and J. R. Hilgard 1975). To the extent that hypnosis and the ritual trance of Thaipusam evoke similar mechanisms, it is likely that the pain control achieved by ritual participants involves perceptual and cognitive changes beyond those evoked by placebos. Of course, as levels of organization in a single biological hierarchy, physiology, and psychology interact, alterations in subjective sensation and level of arousal mediated by endorphins may also lead the person to label his or her mental state as successfully changed and to therefore feel protected from pain and injury.

Are these perceptual and cognitive changes indicative of a profound dissociative state? It is, in fact, not difficult to achieve similar pain control in other settings. For example, it is commonplace in demonstrations of clinical hypnosis to pierce the skin of the hand with a needle, with no pain. Medical students may volunteer to do this with little prompting or training in hypnosis and seem quite surprised when they succeed. Although such pain control is easiest to achieve for individuals high in hypnotic susceptibility (E. R. Hilgard and J. R. Hilgard 1975), in clinical applications in which patient motivation is extremely high, even low levels of hypnotic ability may suffice (Cedercreutz et al. 1978).

It might be protested that a small hypodermic needle is a far cry from the thick spikes and hooks of Thaipusam. What counts in pain perception, though, is not only the size of the injury but its meaning (Melzack and Wall 1982). The injuries incurred during the festival are not punishments or afflictions nor even academic demonstrations; they are celebrations and honors, gifts offered back to the gods in thanks for their help. As such, the injuries are met with positive expectations. Participants may fear the possibility of failing to perform correctly during the ritual more than the potential pain. These social meanings undoubtedly shape the experience of distress in powerful ways.

Thaipusam participants appear to be entranced or transported; they deploy their attention in ways well known to reduce pain experience. Far from maintaining a constant trance state, however, by their own account, participants experience frequent shifts in their attention or degree of absorption during the ritual. When concentration falters and pain intrudes, participants move closer to the drummers and musicians. This provides an external focus of attention that may function as distraction and allows refocusing inward.

Behind the awesome displays of endurance in Thaipusam, then, are social-psychological processes that transform the meaning of events and allow individuals to use ordinary levels of hypnotic capacity to great effect. Ritual trance must be understood as a dynamic process mediated by a wide variety of physical, psychological, and social forces more powerful than the contingencies usually invoked in laboratory settings. It is not easy to isolate these factors in the laboratory or to study their interaction in the field (Ervin et al. 1988).

I have used the example of Thaipusam to emphasize that dissociative phenomena are complex performances, socially shaped, fluctuating over time, and generally not constituted of a single, discrete, and enduring mental state or physiological process. The same point can be made by close examination of the dissociative behavior found in other possession cults (Boddy 1988; Crapanzano and Garrison 1977; Lambek 1989), shamanistic or spiritist healing (Peters and Price-Williams 1983), the posttraumatic stress disorder (PTSD) patient reliving his or her trauma (Young 1990), the DID patient tracing his or her amnesias (Hacking 1991b), or any hypnotic subject engaged in a simple task like arm levitation (McConkey 1991).

Although I have emphasized the intrinsic complexity and diversity of ritual trance, hypnosis, and dissociative phenomena, it is certainly possible to identify areas of overlap and common dimensions. These are best understood, however, not as the *essence* of dissociation but as interacting components of an ongoing process shaped by social context.

For example, as reviewed by Carlson in this volume (see Chapter 3), factor analyses of the Dissociative Experiences Scale (DES; Bernstein and Putnam 1986)—currently the most psychometrically adequate and widely used measure of dissociative phenomena—reveal three dimensions of absorption, perceptual changes, and amnesia. Although these are similar to some items on hypnotizability scales, hypnotic tasks are varied and involve different skills not all of which may be closely related to dissociation (Frankel 1990). Scales for hypnotic susceptibility have few amnesia items and put more emphasis on motor and sensory alterations. Nevertheless, factorial studies of hypnotic susceptibility scales usually reveal at least two basic dimensions: one involving easier items involving imagery or imagination and a second composed of more difficult items, including hallucinations and amnesia (Balthazard and Woody 1985).

It remains unclear to what extent high scores on the DES reflect specific psychopathology, nonspecific distress, or simply normal variations in personality and imagination (Sandberg and Lynn 1992). It is also worth noting that both the DES and current hypnotic susceptibility scales have pools of items that reflect Western cultural and historical notions of the nature of dissociation and hypnosis. Even so, both are multidimensional constructs. A larger pool of items might reveal further dimensions that point more clearly toward latent traits. This possibility is suggested by correlations between the DES or hypnotizability scales and measures of constructs like openness to absorbing experiences (Tellegen and Atkinson 1974), ability to rapidly shift physiological state (Evans 1991), and rapidity or *automaticity* of processing of simple language (Dixon et al. 1990). We will discuss these putative dimensions of hypnotic behavior further in the next section.

STATES OF MIND AND MODES OF DISSOCIATION

It is important to distinguish between dissociation as a behavioral or experiential phenomenon and dissociation as a mental mechanism. In the information-processing metaphors of cognitive psychology, the process of dissociation involves relinquishing executive or self-control of some facet of behavior or experience to a stream of information processing that is not closely identified with the social *I* and that is experienced as involuntary or split off from conscious awareness or recollection. To understand dissociative phenomena, then, we must consider the mechanisms that underlie consciousness as well as those of automatic or nonconscious behavior.

Figure 5–1 displays a simplified heuristic model of four states of mind commonly experienced and some processes that may underlie them (Kirmayer 1992a). There are two conscious states, *self-conscious* or *self-focused awareness* and *unself-conscious awareness;* a preconscious state of daydreaming or *reverie;* and a nonconscious state of automatic or *mindless* behavior *(automaticity).* I use the term *state* here simply to mark off distinctive forms of experience, although I will discuss some of the possible underlying psychological processes later.

Self-consciousness may be directed toward the inner self *(private self-consciousness)* or oneself as a social actor *(public self-consciousness;* Buss 1980). States of high self-consciousness are characterized by conservative cognitive processes aimed at maintaining a coherent sense of self (Gibbons 1990). These have been studied by social psychologists under the rubrics of cognitive dissonance, reactance, and emotional exacerbation (Kirmayer 1990). Self-conscious individuals are engaged in efforts to match their behavior to self-standards and tend to reject suggestions that conflict with their self-standards. Accordingly, they are less likely to respond to suggestions (Gibbons et al. 1979; Scheier et al. 1979). When people are self-conscious

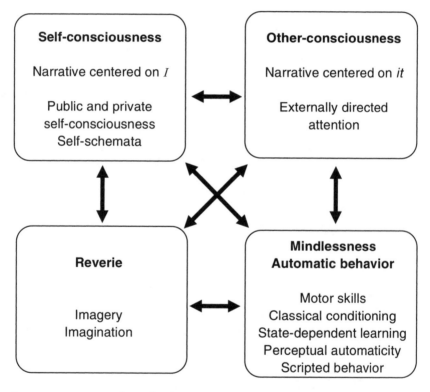

Figure 5–1. States of mind relevant to dissociative experience. Shifts away from self-consciousness may give rise to gaps in experience. In particular, a variety of forms of automatic behavior may give rise to different types of dissociation. *Source.* Reprinted with permission from Kirmayer LJ: "Social Constructions of Hypnosis." *International Journal of Clinical and Experimental Hypnosis* 40:276–300, 1992.

and attribute restrictions on their ability to choose alternatives or take action to others, they may display oppositional behavior.

Much of conscious awareness is not focused on the self but directed toward objects or events that are the content of experience. In this state, people are essentially unaware of the self and more or less absorbed in the external world—even when that world occurs within their own body. This consciousness of the world is, however, easily disrupted whenever a question or reflection causes the person to become aware of his or her self as an observer. In an unself-conscious state, people are less likely to view an attempt to influence or persuade them as infringing on their autonomy. Consequently, when not self-aware, people tend to respond readily to suggestions (Evans 1967). A simple statement that the light in this room is getting brighter, or that the soup is quite salty, will set up expectancies and direct attention in such a way as to alter experience. Such automatic responding to the statements of others as suggestions has adaptive value as a means of rapidly acquiring information or response sets (Schumaker 1991). Most significantly, it serves to create a consensual social reality. The suggestion effect, however, depends crucially on our attitude toward the source of the statements—if we are skeptical, suspicious, or mistrustful, we will be more self-conscious and test each statement against our own critical standards. Response to suggestion will then be diminished. In contrast, settings and cues that shift attention away from the self will result in an increase in response to suggestions. In the case of hypnotic inductions this is further intensified by focusing of attention (Cardeña and Spiegel 1991).

In addition to self-consciousness or instrumental thoughts directed toward the world, people spend a substantial amount of time in daydreaming or *reverie* (Klinger 1978; Singer 1978). Children spend much time absorbed in imagination, but the frequency of reverie diminishes with age (Giambra 1974). In Western societies, formal education and the workplace both devalue daydreaming as a waste of time. As a result, children receive practice in *waking up,* divorcing themselves from their daydreams and reorienting to a consensual reality to engage in task-oriented instrumental behavior. Reverie remains a source of creative, emotion-laden metaphors, images, and ideas (Bachelard 1969). Much of what is called *unconscious* in popular psychology is better understood as reverie that occurs on the fringes of consciousness. Absorption in reverie or daydreaming is often included as a form of dissociative experience.

Finally, despite the illusion we cherish of a continuous stream of conscious awareness, much time is spent in nonconscious, automatic, or mindless behavior (Langer 1989). A great variety of processes underlie such automatic behavior, ranging from simple conditioned responses through the execution of well-practiced motor skills, to complex context-dependent or *scripted* social behaviors (Abelson 1981). Such automatization of skills, habits, and social roles conserves conscious attention and information processing for dealing with novel or unusual situations. We greatly underestimate the amount of our behavior that is determined by such nonconscious automatic processes and the extent to which our conscious accounts are rationalizations after the fact.

Indeed, although psychology tends to personify psychological functions and attribute them to some internal agency, most of our mental faculties do not require awareness or volition, even when they are clearly goal directed. This important distinction between goal-directed and voluntary behavior has been underscored by Bowers (1991). Like breathing, many automatic processes can be consciously redirected or modulated, but under ordinary circumstances they proceed without conscious direction and outside of awareness. For example, in the normal course of events, memories are encoded, stored, and recalled automatically. The encoding and addressing of memories make use of salient cues. When specific cues are present, corresponding memories are evoked. If the cues are absent, we may try to generate them internally in active recall. If we are unable or unwilling to do so, memories will remain inaccessible. From this model, it is a short step to the functional amnesias of hypnosis, in which subjects selectively ignore external and internal cues and so fail to call up recent memories. Clinical dissociative amnesias may, however, be more profound because they involve an additional process of affective state-dependent learning (Reus et al. 1979). Spiegel et al. (1988) have proposed such state-dependent learning as a mechanism in PTSD. Ordinarily, re-evocation of the emotion associated with events serves to facilitate recall (Bower 1981). Trauma-related memories are stored under conditions of very strong emotion. If the emotion is not recreated, the specific memories cannot be recalled. Such affective state-dependent amnesia does not require any active process of avoidance or *amnestic barrier.* If the affect is re-evoked, the traumatic memory may be remembered. Additional cognitive defenses may be employed, however, to avoid re-experiencing such painful affect or to suppress cues that would elicit trauma-related memories.

One form of automaticity with particular relevance to hypnotic and dissociative phenomena is the response to simple language that occurs largely outside of awareness. Recent experiments suggest that *high-hypno-*

tizable subjects differ from control subjects in their perceptual processing (Dixon et al. 1990). Outside the hypnotic situation, high-hypnotizable subjects were found to experience more interference between color and word meaning on the Stroop task (in which subjects must quickly name the color in which color terms are printed [e.g., the word *red* printed in blue letters]). Dixon and colleagues have provided evidence, with tachistoscopic perceptual-masking studies, that this greater interference is due to more rapid processing of the meaning of words by high-hypnotizable subjects. They refer to this as a form of *perceptual automaticity.*

In contrast, Sheehan et al. (1988) found no difference between high and low hypnotic–susceptible subjects in performance on the Stroop task outside of hypnosis. However, in hypnosis, high-susceptible subjects experienced greater interference between color and meaning. When they were given explicit strategies for performing the task (e.g., focusing on a corner of a letter to ignore its shape and just identify the color), high-hypnotizable subjects performed better than *low-hypnotizable* subjects; that is, they showed *less* interference. These findings are remarkable in that performance on the Stroop task has generally been found to be very difficult to modify.

The study by Sheehan and colleagues illustrates the ability of hypnotically susceptible individuals to modify attentional strategies in response to specific instructions given in hypnosis. Whereas the Dixon et al. (1990) study examined only the correlation between the trait of hypnotizability and performance on the Stroop task, the Sheehan study examined the interaction between trait, state (i.e., hypnosis), and instructional set (attentional strategies). The results of the two studies may be reconciled, therefore, if Dixon is right about the trait difference between high- and low-hypnotizable subjects in performance on the Stroop task and if Sheehan is right that hypnotic induction (a state variable) has one effect, whereas specific attentional strategies can have the opposite effect (Dixon and Laurence 1992). In fact, in hypnosis, high-hypnotizable subjects are more able to modify their attentional strategies than low-hypnotizable subjects in response to instructions or social cues. This is an example of a trait-by-state-by-instructional set interaction that illustrates how current research is successfully bridging the artificial dichotomy between state and social-psychological models of hypnosis (Nadon et al. 1991).

These experiments suggest that high-hypnotizable subjects process the meaning of words more quickly than low-hypnotizable subjects. This greater automaticity of language processing might make high-hypnotizable subjects more responsive to suggestions and to the metaphoric implications of words in or out of hypnosis. We will return to this intriguing possibility later in this chapter.

The model of multiple processes underlying states of mind suggests that these four broad states of mind (i.e., self-consciousness, consciousness of the external world, reverie, and automaticity) are not mutually exclusive but reflect the temporary, relative dominance of coexisting or parallel modes of information processing. Any actual state of mind can be viewed as a super-imposition of some degree of activity of each of these modes of information processing. Many different composite states are possible based on different degrees of activation of these modes.

The model of four modes is heterarchical rather than hierarchical. Self-consciousness is not the master mode of cognitive organization or information processing but one among several. Further, changes in state can be seen not as the choice of some executive cognitive agent but as the cooperative effect of parallel modes. These modes may compete for conscious attention at the level of some final common pathway involving a *global workspace* or *working memory* (Dennett 1991; Spiegel 1990). They may also compete for control of motor or action systems. In either case, all modes are at work in the background even when dominated or inhibited by one mode.

We shift rapidly and, for the most part, easily between modes. Because a shift to any mode outside of self-consciousness may be experienced as a rupture in the flow of self-conscious experience, there are a variety of types of dissociation. A shift to unself-conscious awareness is viewed as distraction. A shift to automatic, procedural knowledge is mindlessness (or, if we are adept and retain enough awareness to savor it, *flow;* Csikszentmihalyi 1990). A shift to reverie is absorption and corresponds most closely to hypnotic trance, at least as the concept is employed by many clinicians.

In experimental research, however, hypnosis is studied essentially as what correlates with hypnotic susceptibility (Bowers and Kelly 1979). As we have seen, hypnotizability is factorially complex and includes not only the ability to become absorbed in imagery or imagination but an additional capacity to shift states of mind easily, without interference or intrusion from other modes. In Hilgard's (1977, 1991) neodissociation theory, hypnotizability reflects the ability for subordinate cognitive control systems to escape from conscious control and function autonomously—that is, without interference from conscious awareness, although not without varying degrees of interference from parallel cognitive processes. This capacity for dissociation could reflect differences in dissociability of subordinate cognitive systems, in their responsiveness to evocative stimuli, or in the ability to make a global shift in cognitive organization. The model of four states of mind reflects such global shifts, whereas the various automatic processes to be described are examples of dissociable subsystems of control. For some authors, shifts away from self-consciousness to absorption through externally focused attention or reverie may also be considered forms of dissociation.

As a result of temperament or upbringing, individuals may differ in the tendency for one or another cognitive mode to be dominant and in the fluidity with which they shift between modes (J. R. Hilgard 1970). It is this aspect of psychic organization that allows for a relative dissociation or simultaneous functioning of cognitive modes that is probably most characteristic of high-hypnotizable individuals (E. R. Hilgard 1977). Although hypnosis is not related to sleep, hypnotizability may be related to a general capacity for rapid state changes that includes the ability to fall asleep and wake up easily (Evans 1991). This correlation is found primarily for the amnesia-related items on hypnotizability scales, suggesting that this is separate from the dimension related to imaginative skill.

In sum, hypnotic and dissociative phenomena likely involve the interaction of several distinct psychological processes, including direct suggestibility, imaginative reverie, state-dependent learning, nonconscious modulation of memory and attention, and attribution of action. Contributing to these diverse processes are personality traits involving general features of higher central nervous functioning or cognitive control that influence the changeability and persistence of mental states (Evans 1991) and their propensity to function independently of conscious control (E. R. Hilgard 1977). In the case of hypnosis, these personality traits enhance the ability to direct and focus attention with little effort and to respond to complex stimuli automatically without the interposition or interference of conscious awareness. In the case of dissociative phenomena, these same traits render individuals liable to experiences of involuntariness, alterations of the sense of self, and state-dependent dissociations of memory in response to strong emotion or psychological trauma.

CULTURE AND DISSOCIATIVE EXPERIENCE

On the account sketched in the previous section, our minds are shifty and full of holes, and different forms of dissociation are constant occurrences.

We must work then to close the gaps and mend the ruptures in experience. As Figure 5–2 suggests, we do this in a variety of ways that are hierarchically structured. We shift attention to restore self-consciousness and search for evidence of the causes and consequences of our actions. We review and rehearse memories of events that are initially tied to specific contextual cues and emotions to re-address them in terms of their personal meaning. In this way, memories are woven into a wider associative network so that they can be accessed from many directions. The fragmentary meanings of isolated events are, in turn, woven into narratives that describe our motives, aims, and relationships both in accounts of immediate circumstances and in the longer stories that span a lifetime (Bruner 1990; McAdams 1989). These narratives are then told to others in a process of exchange that solidifies social reality (Bartlett 1932; Kirby 1991).

This hierarchy of ways of weaving together experience works both bottom up and top down. Shifts of attention are governed by the search for salient or recurrent meanings. These meanings, in turn, are based on the narratives by which we identify our selves and our place in the world. These narratives have their origin in the need to give an account of our actions to others and so they depend on socially sanctioned forms of explanation and self-depiction (Howard 1991; Kleinman 1988).

The conscious modes described above are associated with specific types of narrative: self-consciousness with a narrative centered on *I* and contrasting *not-I* or *other,* and consciousness of the world of external objects leading to narratives centered on the third person (i.e., *he, she,* or *it*). Both reverie and automaticity are not conventional narrative modes, although they may influence narrative form. Reverie gives narrative its dream-like associations and poetic texture, whereas automaticity lends to narrative a sense of passivity or inevitability. Narratives are full of metaphors of reverie and automaticity that point toward dissociative processes. But it is the function of self-consciousness to recognize these locutions as just metaphors, to use narrative to keep bridging the dissociative gap, and to weld together a sense of self-continuity and a socially credible personhood. When the metaphors become hypostatized or the narrative falters, we have dissociation.

In this regard, it is interesting that items measuring dissociation on scales like the DES may be taken as either metaphors or as literal descriptions of experience (e.g., "I often feel like I am in a fog"). This seems at first like just a methodological quibble to be resolved by insisting that people endorse items only to the extent they have really experienced them. Re-

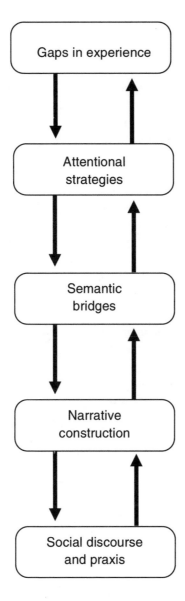

Figure 5–2. The social embedding of dissociative experience. Gaps in experience are smoothed by processes of attention, semantic analysis, narrative construction, and social discourse and praxis. These same processes may, in turn, create dissociative gaps in experience.
Source. Reprinted with permission from Kirmayer LJ: "Social Constructions of Hypnosis." *International Journal of Clinical and Experimental Hypnosis* 40:276–300, 1992.

spondents could be asked, "Do you really mean this or is it just a figure of speech?" Clearly, however, the metaphors for dissociative experience originate in common sensory-perceptual experiences (e.g., being in a fog; Kirmayer 1992b). As noted previously, recent studies suggest that language may be processed more rapidly or automatically in high-hypnotizable individuals. This finding suggests that metaphoric language may have a more direct impact on such individuals in or out of hypnosis. Because metaphors not only express bodily feelings but can evoke them, high-hypnotizable individuals may be more likely to experience changes in sensation, emotion, and cognitive set in response to metaphors generated in their own thoughts or communicated by others. Could the difference between someone who has a dissociative experience, such as depersonalization or derealization, and someone who just says "things seem unreal" to express their sense of existential alienation then be a matter more of degree than kind? People prone to dissociative experience may directly translate metaphors to experience rather than reflectively apprehending metaphor *as* metaphor or philosophical abstraction.

This may also have some bearing on healing ceremonies that appear to involve altered states. The shift in mental state corresponds to a shift in social status or position. We do not know if the apparent dissociations of healer or sufferer are directly related to the physiological or psychological efficacy of the ritual, if any, or primarily serve to mark, in a dramatic fashion, its social significance (Lambek 1989). Whether or not they emphasize an altered state of consciousness, however, healing rituals generally involve a metaphoric journey in which the sufferer's affliction is translated into a new metaphoric world or system of representation (Levi-Strauss 1967). Some move is then made through the metaphoric space and, finally, sufferer and healer are returned to this world where parallel physiological and psychological changes have been effected. If hypnosis or other forms of trance induction serve to intensify the involvement in and impact of metaphoric language, their healing efficacy might be clarified (Kirmayer 1993).

Cultures differ in their tolerance for gaps in narratives, unmotivated events, happenings attributed to extrinsic agencies, and the radical shifts in perspective that accompany shifts in states of mind. Because we are, in fact, constantly experiencing events that cannot be unambiguously assigned to self-directedness or volition, the potential for dissociative attributions and experience is always present. In brief, then, the argument is that gaps in experience are ubiquitous; they are reviewed and woven into narratives by discursive practices. It is the failure of this process of review, semantic bridging, and narrative construction that gives rise to dissociation. If this is so, we understand dissociative phenomena not in terms of a special mental state but as the outcome of an interaction between psychological and social processes.

Culture shapes dissociation through arranging contexts in which imaginative absorption or automaticity is appropriate and can be practiced (Noll 1985), and by providing ethnopsychological concepts of memory and self and modes of narrative reconstruction to describe dissociative experiences. For example, Bateson (1975) describes the socialization for trance of the Balinese, who commonly use trance in the performance of religious arts. A young Balinese dancer is trained by melding her body to her teacher as he moves her like a puppet. She learns to yield control of her body to another in a safe context to achieve a highly valued artistic skill. In this way, involuntariness is given a positive connotation and bodily or procedural knowledge of dancing can be subsequently applied in a state of absorption without conscious direction. This provides a cultural model for forms of motor automaticity akin to the involuntary movements of hypnosis or conversion symptoms.

Similarly, culture may shape amnestic experience. There is considerable evidence that ordinary memory is based on narrative reconstruction (Bartlett 1932; Friedman 1993; Neisser 1982), and, as we have noted, the forms of narrative are cultural conventions (Howard 1991). In societies where time is closely tied to calendar and clock, narratives will commonly anchor events to dates to enhance their credibility, and the preservation of temporal sequence will be an important form of coherence (Munn 1992). In societies where such mechanical time is less important, narratives may take different forms and personal memory will allow for patterns that would appear incoherent or dissociated by the standards of a clockwork society. In fact, few memories are stamped with the time of their occurrence so that the temporal anchors of narratives are largely reconstructions based on contextual cues and conventions (Friedman 1993). Apparent dissociations of experience may then result from different narrative conventions that alter the texture of time.

THE DISINTEGRATION OF IDENTITY

The clinical phenomenology of dissociation includes *derealization, depersonalization, amnesia, identity confusion,* and *identity alteration* (Putnam

1991; Spiegel and Cardeña 1991; Steinberg 1991; Steinberg et al. 1991). These phenomena might arise from disturbances of several discrete psychological processes involving reality testing, body schema, memory, and identity. Alternatively, they can all be understood as consequences of some disruption in the normal integration of experience that establish a stable observing that is rational (monological), univocal, in control, and comfortably embedded in an unquestioned consensual reality. The latter view would make DID the exemplary dissociative disorder, not only because it is the most severe but because it most clearly demonstrates the disturbance of self-organization in dissociation.

The dramatic rise in prevalence of DID in recent years has provoked much controversy about whether DID is being better detected due to refinements in diagnostic criteria and practices, has become more prevalent due to some widespread social problem like child abuse, or is being iatrogenically created in suggestible patients by overly enthusiastic practitioners (Bowers 1991; Fahy 1988; Hacking 1992; Merskey 1992). These alternatives are difficult to resolve, not only because we lack data but because of the imprecision of our notions of personality and dissociation (Hacking 1986; Humphrey and Dennett 1989).

Studies that show high hypnotic susceptibility among DID and dissociative disorder patients also imply that these individuals are highly suggestible (Kluft 1991). This poses a problem for claims that DID patients spontaneously develop their disorder because they would be, on this account, easily shaped by media representations of the disorder or the pointed questions of clinicians. Critics of the rise of DID thus argue that present-day cases are shaped by the mass media and self-help groups.

In a review of published cases of DID, Merskey (1992) could not find a single case in which a pattern of symptoms corresponding to the contemporary condition occurred spontaneously. Many of the classic cases had obvious alternative diagnoses that better fit their symptoms, most often bipolar disorder, cyclothymia, or organic brain syndromes. In several cases, these alternative diagnoses were actually offered by clinicians at the time of the original presentation of the cases. Other cases seemed to involve some form of dissociation, but the appearance of alternate *personalities* was clearly linked to the clinician's explicit instructions to identify and name mood states, ambivalent feelings, or aspects of the self as alternate personalities. Merskey argues that, since the popular book and movie portrayals of multiple personality in the 1950s and 1960s, it is virtually impossible to find cases unaffected by the dramatic media representation of the disorder.

Consequently, there is little or no evidence for the spontaneous production of alter personalities. DID is then largely or wholly a socially constructed disorder.

To the contrary, Spiegel (1988) argues that current multiple personality patients usually have encountered many skeptical physicians prior to their definitive diagnosis so that if their symptomatology were simply a manifestation of suggestibility, they would have long ago abandoned their *alters* in the face of the neglect and outright hostility of skeptical physicians. However, this ignores the fact that suggestions gain power when they are reinforced by social, cultural, and economic factors. Precisely because some clinicians may express renewed interest in working with difficult patients when DID is recognized, this way of expressing distress is likely to be reinforced.

Existing structured interviews and clinical strategies for the diagnosis of DID inevitably introduce implicit or explicit suggestions to identify and personify discrete aspects of the self (Steinberg et al. 1991). Support groups and the growing self-help literature on DID encourage modes of self-understanding and self-depiction, including the use of the pronoun *we* in referring to oneself, that may foster the sense of having multiple selves in vulnerable individuals (see, for example, Cohen et al. 1991). However, it is incontestable that patients respond differently to these prompts. Some offer detailed accounts of their own spontaneous dissociative experiences and apparent changes in personality, whereas others find the questions difficult to understand or purely metaphorical in nature. Whatever their nosological implications, these differences require explanations beyond suggestion or modeling.

Many new cases of DID come from the ranks of those previously diagnosed with borderline personality disorder (BPD), and, like BPD patients, they may have received numerous other diagnoses in the past (Kluft 1991). BPD patients are prone to dissociative experiences (Zanarini et al. 1990). Zweig-Frank et al. (in press) found that BPD patients had significantly higher DES scores (mean = 24.8 ± 15.2) than a comparison group of patients with other personality disorders (mean = 13.2 ± 10.2, t = 5.6, P < .001). These patients, along with others with less severe psychopathology, may tend to experience their own states of mind and aspects of the self as split-off entities and, with little prompting, speak of them in the third person or otherwise reify them as autonomous agents (Benner and Joscelyne 1984; Peters 1988).

The ease with which some patients personify aspects of themselves and experience functional amnesias may reflect personality traits or psycho-pathological processes that cut across other diagnostic categories. Lynn and Rhue (1988) have studied individuals high in hypnotic ability whom they term *fantasy-prone personalities*. Depending on coexisting pathology, these individuals may experience their hypnotic or dissociative experiences as useful skills or as worrisome symptoms. When combined with affective instability and identity confusion, this trait could give rise to many of the features of DID. In particular, split-off aspects of the self associated with intense affect or unacceptable trauma memories or experiences could inter-act with hypnotic ability to give rise to personified aspects of the self. The problem with calling each of these modes of expression *personalities* is that an ordinary personality is, in fact, made up of ambivalences, contradictions, and a plurality of narrative voices in dialogue, argument, and negotiation within the self (Gagnon 1992; Watkins 1986). This is the stuff of most depth psychologies.

As discussed in the previous section of this chapter, many philosophers and psychologists have come to view the self as a narrative construction (Bruner 1990; Howard 1991; Kirby 1991; McAdams 1989; Ricouer 1992; Sarbin 1986). From this perspective, the self is a coherent story we construct about our actions, and the *I* is the narrative *center of gravity* in our story (Dennett 1991). When multiple stories are created, with different narrative centers, we may have multiple selves (Humphrey and Dennett 1989). This perspective suggests the importance for conceptions of dissociation of un-derstanding the relationship of narrative construction to emotion, memory, and the sense of self.

Examining the scientific literature, Hacking (1992) identified four suc-cessive waves of interest in multiple personality. From about 1800 onward, there were sporadic reports of *double-consciousness* in European and American medical literature (Hacking 1991c). The term *personality* began to be applied to similar changes in consciousness from 1875 in France, when several cases of *dual personality* were described. This was followed by a period of great interest in the United States that lasted until the early part of the twentieth century (Carlson 1981; Hacking 1991b). The most recent wave began in the 1970s and by 1982 was described as an epidemic (Boor 1982).

Hacking (1992) argues that each wave of popularity of the diagnosis of DID was made possible by its linkage with some social issue of great sa-lience and importance. In the first American wave, it was the influence of spiritualism and its quasi-scientific partner, spiritism, that encouraged the emergence of the multiple personalities that captivated William James, Morton Prince, and their contemporaries (Kenny 1986; Prince 1905/1978). Reports of multiple personality waned with the rise of scientific rationality as the language of self-depiction. The remarkable boom in the diagnosis of DID in the last two decades has been linked with the recognition of the widespread existence of severe child abuse, which is generally viewed as an important causal factor in DID (Hacking 1991a; 1992).

Proponents of DID as a distinct entity tend to see a direct link between childhood trauma and the creation of alternate personalities that may be recognized spontaneously or under careful clinical inquiry (Kluft 1991). Criticism of the nature of DID may then be perceived as an attack on the reality and prevalence of child abuse. However, the correlation of child abuse with dissociative experience does not demonstrate a simple causal link. Other factors, including temperament and family pathology, may contribute to the high prevalence of dissociative experiences in abuse victims (Nash et al. 1993). Critics may acknowledge both the reality of child abuse and its association with dissociative phenomena or disorders but see the specific feature of multiplicity as an imaginative fabrication that occurs largely after the fact.

The amnestic barriers or dissociations of separate strands of memory associated with different personalities are usually traced back to severe traumas that prompted the splitting or dissociation as an adaptive strategy for escape from an inescapable situation (Kluft 1991). The evidence for these traumas may be clear memories or vague recollections associated with vivid bodily sensations and fragmentary images (Frankel 1993). Memory for traumatic experiences is not necessarily either more or less accurate than memory for less emotionally charged events (Christianson 1992). The one consistent effect of trauma or emotional intensity on memory is a narrowing of attention during registration such that many details may not be noticed. This could give rise to difficulties in recovering memories due to a lack of contextual information (Spiegel 1990).

However, work on the psychology of memory suggests that most personal, autobiographical memory is not based on veridical snapshots of experiences but is a narrative reconstruction that responds as much to current context of recall as it does to past events (Bartlett 1932; Frankel 1993; Friedman 1993; Neisser 1982). Hence, our personal history is highly changeable according to current circumstances. To the extent that the sense of self depends on the stories we construct and tell about ourselves—and these stories, in turn, depend on a fallible and mutable memory open to social influence—the sense of self is equally mutable, changeable, and socially constructed.

Multiple personality is, at present, largely a North American phenomena, although recent series of cases have been reported from Europe (Boon and Draijer 1993; Modestin 1992) and Japan (Takahashi 1990). In many other cultures, alternate persons or changes in personality commonly appear in the context of spirit possession (Adityanjee et al. 1989; Bourguignon 1967; Kenny 1981). These persons, however, represent culturally identified beings—ancestors, spirits, or gods—and not the idiosyncratic childhood of the individual. Far from being pathological, the experience and expression of multiple voices within the person most often have positive religious, healing, and esthetic value (Boddy 1988; Crapanzano and Garrison 1977; Leavitt 1993). Some form of overarching integration is provided by the social system that assigns culturally appropriate and intelligible roles and identities to the inhabiting spirits. The plural voices of the self are then contained by a larger social order.

In religious possession cults, the other is not primarily a feared and intrusive presence but a holy visitation to be received and welcomed. Thus the first intimations of the god's presence lead the person to relinquish control, to let self-consciousness subside, and, afterward, to attribute actions to the inspiriting other. In fact, the cultural use of the idiom of possession often does not involve any actual dissociative experience. Its crucial aspect resides in attributing actions to the possessing god and the physical and social embodiment of that god's identity (Lambek 1989).

Krippner (1987) described how Brazilian spiritist practices may provide a social arena for the expression and regulation of pathology similar to DID. However, as Bourguignon (1989) notes, although there may be psychological similarities between the possession experiences of Umbandista in Brazil and the multiple personality patient in North America, the fact that in the former case the alters are demons or gods to be either exorcised or domesticated, whereas in the latter they are fragments of the self to be reintegrated leads to fundamentally different natural histories of dissociation.

The participant in a possession cult, often an oppressed woman with few options for protest, gains social support from the cult and, through the voice of the god who possesses her (and who she, of course, also possesses), a means of demanding redress within her family and society (Lambek 1989; Lewis 1971). The cultural idiom of possession then provides a socially sanctioned means of protest and contestation. Similarly, the rise of DID can be seen not only in terms of individual psychopathology but as the emergence of a new form of social protest against the brutalization and oppression of women and children.

DID has other social precursors in Western folk psychology, however, that set it apart from dissociative disorders in other cultures. The unity of the person assumed by folk psychology is something of an exaggeration. We are different people in different situations and many other cultures readily acknowledge this by subordinating the concept of the person as self-directed individual to his or her social role, context, or current circumstances (Ross and Nisbett 1991; Shweder 1991). In contrast, the Western univocal person must constantly strive to reconcile or rationalize inconsistencies and lacunae in his or her behavior across situations (Kirmayer 1989). If multivocality is intrinsic to the human condition, then the Western person is engaged in a constant process of minimizing or subduing alternate voices.

The self accessed in self-conscious awareness is itself a culturally constructed schema that includes values, ideals, and standards against which behavior is judged and controlled (Markus and Kitayama 1991). These standards may include various degrees of tolerance for other modes of unselfconscious awareness or automaticity. Based on this evaluation of other states of mind, the self-conscious mode may attempt to suppress or subvert other modes. But as we have seen, reverie, automaticity, and externally oriented consciousness have their own ways of intruding, not least because each is the most effective means of coping with some situations.

People in other cultures are more comfortable acknowledging the limitations of self-consciousness and the fluidity of the self (Leavitt 1993). In Western Protestant societies, however, self-direction and self-control have long been marks of distinction, central to our concepts of health and moral rectitude (Weisz et al. 1984). This emphasis on conscious, rational, personal choice in accounts of our motives and actions sits uneasily with the evidence of unconscious, social, and biological processes that govern much of our behavior (Rorty 1985). In particular, it ignores the central role of imaginative life in the integration of the person (Watkins 1986).

It is in this cultural context that we can understand the history of multiple personality as a culture-specific dissociative disorder (Kenny 1981). DID can be understood as a concretization or literalism in the imaginative and symbolic life of the self. The DID patient suffers from the exaggerated individualism or narcissism of North American culture that leads many to feel a lack of a unifying self, a sense of emptiness, incompleteness, a "center that will not hold" (Bellah et al. 1985; Cushman 1990). The alters of the DID patient are drawn from personal history and so affirm individualism in their apparent idiosyncrasy, even if, in fact, their characteristics and roles are highly stereotyped. In contemporary North America, there is no overarching collective myth to integrate the voices into a larger whole, so a personal myth must be constructed through the medium of psychotherapy (Kirmayer 1993). The therapeutic treatment of DID encourages the patient to adopt many voices and so to discover in the gaps of dissociation the hidden richness of the plural self (Samuels 1989). In the absence of communal or religious rituals to embody and give voice to this plurality, North Americans who have had their inner voices violently suppressed must resort to the private suffering of dissociative disorders or the public exculpation of the new psychotherapies of dissociation.

For some clinicians, the fact that patients previously given other diagnoses now are found to have DID is a demonstration of progress in nosology and diagnostic interviewing brought about by a reconceptualization of the role of dissociation in psychopathology. For others this rediagnosis and re-reorientation of treatment is misleading and runs the risk of aggravating the patient's condition by excessive attention to split-off aspects of the self (Chodoff 1987). In the absence of controlled clinical trials, opinions about optimal treatment reflect not only clinical wisdom but cultural concepts of personhood, moral agency, and the nature of imagination (Halleck 1990).

CONCLUSION

Dissociation involves a gap or disturbance in normal patterns of integration of memory, self, and perception. We recognize this disruption against standards we have for the continuity, univocality, and rationality of the self. This is expressed in a temporal narrative centered on rational motives for our actions and responses. This depiction of the self is, to some extent, culture bound. People in other cultures do not demand the same amount of continuity, consistency, univocality, or rationality in behavior. Ignoring this may lead us to pathologize experiences like possession, which represent a socially sanctioned solution for problems rather than an illness or disorder. It may also lead us to miss other forms of pathology that involve univocality or excessive rationality in contexts where these are socially inappropriate. It is this univocality that leads patients to describe spontaneous thoughts and feelings on a continuum from *I* to *it*. Too much *I* can be as much a problem, in some societies, as too much *it* is in our own. Cultural concepts of remembering and forgetting, time, and memory shape the narrative accounts of actions and experience and may make dissociations more common and less pathological than they are held to be in current nosology. In cultures where not knowing, not remembering, and involuntariness are socially sanctioned or normative, apparent dissociative episodes may be incorrectly diagnosed on the basis of simple disavowal without any psychopathological significance.

In arguing for this social perspective, I do not mean to question the existence of clinical dissociative phenomena but to show their relationship to the psychology of everyday life. In my experience, dissociative phenomena are often subtle, delicate, and involve the interaction of ordinary cognitive and social processes related to imagination and self-characterization through memory and narrative. The extreme cases—like DID—may exhibit unique features, but they are certainly not the only phenomena of clinical interest, nor is it certain that they are discontinuous with or unrelated to the milder more common phenomena. They may seem more dramatic because of other personality characteristics of the patients (e.g., histrionic style) or the urgency with which they seek to convey their distress, which may have been dismissed by others (Spiegel 1988).

Indeed, this dismissal by some clinicians occurs in part because of cultural ideas about the self that make it hard to accept the plurality of voices and autonomous psychological processes within the person. The fascination with dissociation in contemporary psychiatry reflects decades of relative neglect, but even more it stems from the fact that certain folk psychological ideas about the self are violated by dissociative phenomena. The Western self nurtures the fantasy that it is the master of all it surveys. This monolithic version of the self may be a cultural fiction that is wearing thin.

REFERENCES

Abelson RP: Psychological status of the script concept. Am Psychol 36:715–729, 1981

Adityanjee RGSP, Kandewal SS: Current status of multiple personality in India. Am J Psychiatry 146:1607–1610, 1989

Bachelard G: The Poetics of Reverie. Boston, MA, Beacon Press, 1969

Balthazard CG, Woody EZ: The "stuff" of hypnotic performance: a review of psychometric approaches. Psychol Bull 98:283–296, 1985

Barber J, Mayer D: Evaluation of the efficacy and neural mechanism of a hypnotic analgesia procedure in experimental and clinical dental pain. Pain 4:41–48, 1977

Bartlett FC: Remembering. Cambridge, MA, Cambridge University Press, 1932

Bateson G: Some components of socialization for trance. Ethos 3:143–155, 1975

Bellah RN, Madsen R, Sullivan WM, et al: Habits of the Heart: Individualism and Commitment in American Life. Berkeley, University of California Press, 1985

Benner DG, Joscelyne B: Multiple personality as a borderline disorder. J Nerv Ment Dis 172:98–104, 1984

Bernstein E, Putnam F: Development, reliability and validity of a dissociation scale. J Nerv Ment Dis 174:727–735, 1986

Boddy J: Spirits and selves in Northern Sudan: the cultural therapeutics of possession and trance. American Ethnologist 15:4–27, 1988

Boon S, Draijer N: Multiple personality disorder in The Netherlands: a clinical investigation of 71 patients. Am J Psychiatry 150:489–494, 1993

Boor M: The multiple personality epidemic: additional cases and inferences regarding diagnosis, etiology, dynamics, and treatment. J Nerv Ment Dis 170:302–304, 1982

Bourguignon E: World distribution and patterns of possession states, in Trance and Possession States. Edited by Prince R. Montreal, Canada, RM Bucke Society, 1967, pp 3–34

Bourguignon E: Multiple personality, possession trance, and the psychic unity of mankind. Ethos 17:371–384, 1989

Bower GH: Mood and memory. Am Psychol 36:129–148, 1981

Bowers KS: Dissociation in hypnosis and multiple personality disorder. Int J Clin Exp Hypn 39:155–176, 1991

Bowers KS, Kelly P: Stress, disease, psychotherapy, and hypnosis. J Abnorm Psychol 88:490–505, 1979

Bruner J: Acts of Meaning. Cambridge, MA, Harvard University Press, 1990

Buss AH: Self-Consciousness and Social Anxiety. San Francisco, CA, WH Freeman, 1980

Cardeña E, Spiegel D: Suggestibility, absorption, and dissocation: an integrative model of hypnosis, in Human Suggestibility: Advances in Theory, Research, and Application. Edited by Schumaker JF. London, Routledge, 1991, pp 93–107

Carlson ET: The history of multiple personality in the United States; I: the beginnings. Am J Psychiatry 138:666–668, 1981

Cedercreutz C, Lähteenmäki R, Tulikoura J: Hypnotic treatment of headache and vertigo in skull injured patients. Int J Clin Exp Hypn 24:195–201, 1978

Chaves J: Pain control, in Hypnosis: The Cognitive-Behavioral Perspective. Edited by Spanos NP, Chaves JF. Buffalo, NY, Prometheus Press, 1989

Chodoff P: Multiple personality disorder (letter). Am J Psychiatry 144:124, 1987

Christianson S-A: Emotional stress and eyewitness memory: a critical review. Psychol Bull 112:284–309, 1992

116

Cohen BM, Giller E, Lynn W: Multiple Personality Disorder From the Inside Out. Baltimore, MD, Sidran Press, 1991

Crapanzano V, Garrison V: Case Studies in Spirit Possession, New York, Wiley, 1977

Csikszentmihalyi M: Flow: The Psychology of Optimal Experience. New York, Harper, 1990

Cushman P: Why the self is empty: toward a historically situated psychology. Am Psychol 45:599–611, 1990

Dennett DC: Consciousness Explained. Boston, MA, Little, Brown, 1991

Dixon M, Laurence J-R: Hypnotic susceptibility and verbal automaticity: automatic and strategic processing differences in the Stroop color-naming task. J Abnorm Psychol 101:344–347, 1992

Dixon M, Brunet A, Laurence J-R: Hypnotizability and automaticity: toward a parallel distributed processing model of hypnotic responding. J Abnorm Psychol 99:336–343, 1990

Ervin FR, Palmour RM, Pearson Murphy BE, et al: The psychobiology of trance; II: physiological and endocrine correlates. Transcultural Psychiatric Research Review 25:267–284, 1988

Evans FJ: Suggestibility in the normal waking state. Psychol Bull 67:114–129, 1967

Evans FJ: Expectancy, therapeutic instructions, and the placebo response, in Placebo: Theory, Research, and Mechanisms. Edited by White L, Tursky B, Schwartz GE. New York, Guilford, 1985, pp 215–228

Evans FJ: Hypnotizability: individual differences in dissociation and the flexible control of psychological processes, in Theories of Hypnosis: Current Models and Perspectives. Edited by Lynn SJ, Rhue JW. New York, Guilford, 1991, pp 144–168

Fahy TA: The diagnosis of multiple personality disorder: a critical review. Br J Psychiatry 153:597–606, 1988

Frankel FH: Hypnotizability and dissociation. Am J Psychiatry 147:823–829, 1990

Frankel FH: Adult reconstructions of childhood events in the multiple personality literature. Am J Psychiatry 150:954–958, 1993

Friedman WJ: Memory for the time of past events. Psychol Bull 113:44–66, 1993

Gagnon JH: The self, its voices, and their discord, in Investigating Subjectivity. Edited by Ellis C, Flaherty MG. Newbury Park, CA, Sage, 1992, pp 221–243

Giambra LM: Daydreaming across the life span: late adolescent to senior citizen. Int J Aging Hum Dev 5:115–140, 1974

Gibbons FX: Self-attention and behavior: a review and theoretical update, in Advances in Experimental Social Psychology. Edited by Zana M. San Diego, CA, Academic Press 1990, pp 249–304

Gibbons FX, Carver CS, Scheier MF, et al: Self-focused attention and the placebo effect: fooling some of the people some of the time. Journal of Experimental Social Psychology 15:263–274, 1979

Glover H: Emotional numbing: a possible endorphin-mediated phenomenon associated with post-traumatic stress disorders and other allied psychopathologic states. Journal of Traumatic Stress 5:643–675, 1992

Hacking I: Making up people, in Reconstructing Individualism: Autonomy, Individuality, and the Self in Western Thought. Edited by Heller T, Sosner M, Wellberry D. Stanford, CA, Stanford University Press, 1986, pp 222–236

Hacking I: The making and molding of child abuse. Critical Inquiry 17:253–288, 1991a

Hacking I: Two souls in one body. Critical Inquiry 17:838–867, 1991b

Hacking I: Double consciousness in Britain 1815–1875. Dissociation 4:134–146, 1991c

Hacking I: Multiple personality disorder and its hosts. History of the Human Sciences 5:3–31, 1992

Halleck SL: Dissociative phenomena and the question of responsibility. Int J Clin Exp Hypn 38:298–314, 1990

Hilgard ER: Divided Consciousness: Multiple Controls in Human Thought and Action. New York, Wiley, 1977

Hilgard ER: A neodissociation interpretation of hypnosis, in Theories of Hypnosis: Current Models and Perspectives. Edited by Lynn SJ, Rhue JW. New York, Guilford, 1991, pp 83–104

Hilgard ER, Hilgard JR: Hypnosis in the Relief of Pain. San Francisco, CA, Kauffman, 1975

Hilgard JR: Personality and Hypnosis: A Study of Imaginative Involvement. Chicago, IL, University of Chicago Press, 1970

Howard GS: Culture tales: a narrative approach to thinking, cross-cultural psychology, and psychotherapy. Am Psychol 46:187–197, 1991

Humphrey N, Dennett D: Speaking for ourselves: an assessment of multiple personality disorder. Raritan: A Quarterly Review 9:68–98, 1989

Kenny MG: Multiple personality and spirit possession. Psychiatry 44:337–358, 1981

Kenny MG: The Passion of Ansel Bourne: Multiple Personality in American Culture. Washington, DC, Smithsonian Institution Press, 1986

Kirby AP: Narrative and the Self. Bloomington, IN, Indiana University Press, 1991

Kirmayer LJ: Psychotherapy and the cultural concept of the person. Santé, Culture, Health 6:241–270, 1989

Kirmayer LJ: Resistance, reactance and reluctance to change: a cognitive attributional approach to strategic interventions. Journal of Cognitive Psychotherapy 4:83–104, 1990

Kirmayer LJ: Social constructions of hypnosis. Int J Clin Exp Hypn 40:276–300, 1992a

Kirmayer LJ: The body's insistence on meaning: metaphor as presentation and representation in illness experience. Med Anthropol 6:323–346, 1992b

Kirmayer LJ: Healing and the invention of metaphor: the effectiveness of symbols revisited. Culture, Medicine, and Psychiatry 17:161–195, 1993

Kleinman A: The Illness Narratives. New York, Basic Books, 1988

Klinger E: Modes of normal conscious flow, in The Stream of Consciousness. Edited by Pope KS, Singer JL. New York, Plenum, 1978, pp 226–258

Kluft R: Multiple personality disorder, in American Psychiatric Press Review of Psychiatry, Vol 10. Edited by Tasman A, Goldfinger SM. Washington, DC, American Psychiatric Press, 1991, pp 161–188

Krippner S: Cross-cultural approaches to multiple personality disorder: practices in Brazilian spiritism. Ethos 15:273–295, 1987

Lambek M: From disease to discourse: remarks on the conceptualization of trance and spirit possession, in Altered States of Consciousness and Mental Health: A Cross-Cultural Perspective. Edited by Ward CA. London, Sage, 1989, pp 36–61

Langer EJ: Mindfulness. Reading, MA, Addison-Wesley, 1989

Leavitt J: Are trance and possession disorders? Transcultural Psychiatric Research Review 30:51–57, 1993

Levine JD, Gordon NC, Fields HL: The mechanism of placebo analgesia. Lancet 2:654–657, 1978

Levi-Strauss C: Structural Anthropology. New York, Basic Books, 1967

Lewis IM: Ecstatic Religion: An Anthropological Study of Spirit Possession and Shamanism. Middlesex, UK, Penguin, 1971

Lynn SJ, Rhue JW: Fantasy proneness: hypnosis, developmental antecedents, and psychopathology. Am Psychol 43:35–44, 1988

Markus HR, Kitayama S: Culture and the self: implications for cognition, emotion, and motivation. Psychol Rev 98:224–253, 1991

McAdams DP: The development of a narrative identity, in Personality Psychology: Recent Trends and Emerging Directions. Edited by Buss DM, Cantor N. New York, Springer-Verlag, 1989, pp 160–174

McConkey KM: The construction and resolution of experience and behavior in hypnosis, in Theories of Hypnosis: Current Models and Perspectives. Edited by Lynn SJ, Rhue JW. New York, Guilford, 1991, pp 542–563

McGlashan TH, Evans FJ, Orne MT: The nature of hypnotic analgesia and placebo response to experimental pain. Psychosom Med 31:227–246, 1969

Melzack R, Wall P: The Challenge of Pain. Middlesex, UK, Penguin, 1982

Merskey HM: The manufacture of personalities: the production of multiple personality disorder. Br J Psychiatry 160:327–340, 1992

Modestin J: Multiple personality disorder in Switzerland. Am J Psychiatry 149:88–92, 1992

Munn ND: The cultural anthropology of time: a critical essay. Annual Review of Anthropology 21:93–123, 1992

Nadon R, Laurence J-R, Perry C: The two disciplines of scientific hypnosis: a synergistic model, in Theories of Hypnosis: Current Models and Perspectives. Edited by Lynn SJ, Rhue JW. New York, Guilford, 1991, pp 485–519

Nash MR, Hulsey TL, Sexton MC, et al: Long-term sequelae of childhood sexual abuse: perceived family environment, psychopathology, and dissociation. J Consult Clin Psychol 61:276–283, 1993

Neisser U: Memory Observed: Remembering in Natural Contexts. San Francisco, CA, WH Freeman, 1982

Noll R: Mental imagery cultivation as a cultural phenomenon: the role of visions in shamanism. Current Anthropology 26:443–461, 1985

Orne MT: On the social psychology of the psychological experiment: with particular reference to demand characteristics and their implications. Am Psychol 17:776–783, 1962

Peters LG: Borderline personality disorder and the possession syndrome: an ethnopsychoanalytic perspective. Transcultural Psychiatric Research Review 25:5–46, 1988

Peters LG, Price-Williams DG: A phenomenological overview of trance. Transcultural Psychiatric Research Review 20:5–39, 1983

Prince M: The Dissociation of a Personality: The Hunt for the Real Miss Beauchamp (1905). Oxford, Oxford University Press, 1978

Putnam FW: Dissociative phenomena, in American Psychiatric Press Review of Psychiatry, Vol 10. Edited by Tasman A, Goldfinger SM. Washington, DC, American Psychiatric Press, 1991, pp 145–160

Reus VI, Weingarten H, Post RM: Clinical implications of state-dependent learning. Am J Psychiatry 136:927–932, 1979

Ricoeur P: Oneself as Another. Chicago, IL, University of Chicago Press, 1992

Rorty AO: Self-deception, akrasia, and irrationality, in The Multiple Self. Edited by Elster J. Cambridge, Cambridge University Press, 1985, pp 115–131

Ross L, Nisbett RE: The Person and the Situation: Perspectives of Social Psychology. Philadelphia, PA, Temple Univeristy Press, 1991

Samuels A: The Plural Psyche: Personality, Morality and the Father. London, Routledge, 1989

Sandberg DA, Lynn SJ: Dissociative experiences, psychopathology and adjustment, and child and adolescent maltreatment in female college students. J Abnorm Psychol 101:717–723, 1992

Sarbin TR (ed): Narrative Psychology: The Storied Nature of Human Conduct. New York, Praeger, 1986

Sarbin TR: The construction and reconstruction of hypnosis, in Hypnosis: The Cognitive-Behavioral Perspective. Edited by Spanos NP, Chaves JF. Buffalo, NY, Prometheus, 1989, pp 400–416

Scheier MF, Carver CS, Gibbons FX: Self-directed attention, awareness of bodily states, and suggestibility. J Pers Soc Psychol 37:1576–1588, 1979

Schumaker JF: The adaptive value of suggestibility and dissociation, in Human Suggestibility: Advances in Theory, Research, and Application. Edited by Schumaker JF. London, Routledge, 1991, pp 108–131

Sheehan PW, Donovan P, MacLeod CM: Strategy manipulation and the Stroop effect in hypnosis. J Abnorm Psychol 97:455–460, 1988

Shweder R: Thinking Through Culture: Expeditions in Cultural Psychology. Cambridge, MA, Harvard University Press, 1991

Simons RC, Pfaff G: Floating in the Air, Followed by the Wind. Bloomington, IN, Indiana University Audio-Visual Center, 1973

Simons RC, Ervin FR, Prince RH: The psychobiology of trance; I: training for Thaipusam. Transcultural Psychiatric Research Review 25:249–266, 1988

Singer JL: Experimental studies of daydreaming and the stream of thought, in The Stream of Consciousness. Edited by Pope KS, Singer JL. New York, Plenum, 1978, pp 187–225

Spanos N: Hypnotic behavior: a social-psychological interpretation of amnesia, analgesia, and "trance logic." The Behavioral and Brain Sciences 9:449–502, 1986

Spiegel D: The treatment accorded those who treat patients with multiple personality disorder. J Nerv Ment Dis 176:535–536, 1988

Spiegel D: Hypnosis, dissociation, and trauma: hidden and overt observers, in Repression and Dissociation: Implications for Personality Theory, Psychopathology, and Health. Edited by Singer JL. Chicago, IL, University of Chicago Press, 1990, pp 121–142

Spiegel D, Cardeña E: Disintegrated experience: the dissociative disorders revisited. J Abnorm Psychol 100:366–378, 1991

Spiegel D, Hunt T, Dondershine HE: Dissociation and hypnotizability in posttraumatic stress disorder. Am J Psychiatry 145:301–305, 1988

Steinberg M: The spectrum of depersonalization: assessment and treatment, in American Psychiatric Press Review of Psychiatry, Vol 10. Edited by Tasman A, Goldfinger SM. Washington, DC, American Psychiatric Press, 1991, pp 223–247

Steinberg M, Rounsaville B, Cicchetti D: Detection of dissociative disorders in psychiatric patients by a screening instrument and a structured diagnostic interview. Am J Psychiatry 148:1050–1054, 1991

Takahashi Y: Is multiple personality disorder really rare in Japan? Dissociation 3:57–59, 1990

Tellegen A, Atkinson G: Openness to absorbing and self-altering experiences ("absorption"): a trait related to hypnotic susceptibility. J Abnorm Psychol 83:268–277, 1974

Watkins M: Invisible Guests: The Development of Imaginal Dialogues. Hillsdale, NJ, Analytic Press, 1986

Weisz JR, Rothbaum FM, Blackburn TC: Standing out and standing in: the psychology of control in America and Japan. Am Psychol 39:955–969, 1984

Willer JC, Dehen H, Cambier J: Stress-induced analgesia in humans: endogenous opioids and naloxone-reversible depression of pain reflexes. Science 212:689–691, 1981

Young A: Moral conflicts in a psychiatric hospital treating combat-related PTSD, in Social Science Perspectives on Medical Ethics. Edited by Weiss G. Boston, MA, Kluwer, 1990, pp 65–82

Zanarini MC, Gunderson JG, Frankenburg FR, et al: Discriminating borderline personality disorder from other Axis II disorders. Am J Psychiatry 147:161–167, 1990

Zweig-Frank H, Paris J, Guzder J: Dissociation in borderline and non-borderline personality disorders. Journal of Personality Disorders (in press)

CHAPTER 6

Culture and Dissociation: A Comparison of *Ataque de Nervios* Among Puerto Ricans and Possession Syndrome in India

Roberto Lewis-Fernández, M.D.

The search for the brain-mind mechanism(s) of dissociation is complicated by enduring uncertainty, despite decades of research, over whether the tremendous diversity of recorded trances and altered states derive from one, a few, or multiple neuropsychological processes (see Erdelyi, Chapter 1, this volume). Even within a single cultural group, United States Euro-Americans, there are multiple normative sequences of behavior and experience—*normal* and *pathological, secular* and *religious*—that are characterized by significant alterations of consciousness, memory, or identity and thus appear dissociative in origin. These include hypnosis, dissociative identity disorder (DID; formerly called multiple personality disorder), some forms of meditation, conversion reactions, Pen-

This chapter was supported by a Dupont-Warren Psychiatry Fellowship at Harvard Medical School (1990–1991), by National Institute of Mental Health fellowship in clinically relevant medical anthropology RER-2 5 T32 MH18006-07 (1991–1993), by the MacArthur Foundation Research Network on Mind-Body Interactions, and by the Nathan Cummings Foundation. I thank Arthur Kleinman, David Spiegel, Mitchell Weiss, Peter Guarnaccia, Byron Good, Goretti Almeida, and the Dissociation Group and Medical Anthropology Fellows at Harvard University.

tecostal glossolalia, dissociative (psychogenic) amnesia, *channeling,* post-traumatic stress disorder, charismatic healing, and fugue, among others. Historically, this number is supplemented by important dissociative philosophic and religious practices—such as spiritualistic séances and automatic writing in New England and elsewhere in the United States, Swedenborgian mysticism, snake handling, and Shaker dancing (Brown 1970; Goodman 1988; Gurney et al. 1918; James 1986)—as well as by several dissociative afflictions no longer presenting frequently in this population—such as somnambulism, hysterical *crises,* and demonic possession (Carlson 1986; Ellenberger 1970; Janet 1907/1965). This diversity of forms increases exponentially when we admit evidence from the worldwide cross-cultural record, where culturally authorized dissociation is markedly more prevalent than in the United States. Does this multiplicity of trances and altered states represent differentiations from a unitary (or a discrete number) of universal brain-mind processes? Or, instead, is it the result of the convergence of many distinct neuropsychological mechanisms into a finite number of locally patterned dissociative final common pathways? In either case, what is the role played by the indigenous culture in the configuration of these normative behavioral-experiential dissociative sequences?

Any investigation attempting to discover the brain-mind mechanism(s) of dissociation must come to grips with these dilemmas. It is not enough to simplify the problem by mooting the question of cultural patterning in the name of a postulated neuropsychological universalism (which itself is far from certain) nor even to select a culturally homogeneous study sample in the hope of controlling for cultural variance. Rather than clarify the issue, these research methods would tend to obscure it by implying that it is possible to isolate (or ignore) culture as a variable in the study of human experience. According to this view, culture is the lens through which *others* see the world; our outlook is "natural." Culture, instead, should be problematized in the research methodology; evoking its central role in the patterning of experience should be essential to our investigation. All humans encode their experience after the collective categories of the cultural world to which they belong. As a result, individual experiences will tend to be bound within the cultural norms from which they arise, which structure their phenomenology, interpretation, distribution of setting and sequence, and association with other units of experience. A clear understanding of the patterns imposed by this cultural grid on the structure of individual experience is necessary if we are to discover the contribution to this structure of underlying neuropsychological substrates.

Disentangling these factors becomes very difficult unless we include in our investigation the experiences of diverse cultural groups. If we do not, we risk interpreting the neuropsychological expressions of particular cultural constructions as the singular brain-mind mechanisms of the human race. But if we take a comparatist perspective and examine the experiences of multiple cultures with regard to a specific realm of human activity, such as dissociation (paying as much attention to differences as to similarities), we would be able to catalogue a variety of relationships between cultural constructions and neuropsychological mechanisms. We could observe the full range of brain-mind processes mediating the various cultural forms of dissociation and thus come closer to resolving the dilemma posed earlier of divergent universalism versus convergent particularism.

CROSS-CULTURAL STUDY OF DISSOCIATION

The cross-cultural record contains an extremely diverse collection of locally patterned dissociative experiences.[1] Globally, a majority of these states are considered normal in their indigenous cultural settings inasmuch as they do not lead to distress or impairment, they arise in willing subjects in appropriate and usually religious contexts, and they are often experienced as beneficial. Few dissociative states are labeled indigenously as illnesses. These states usually recur involuntarily or in inappropriate forms or settings, they cause distress or impairment, and they are frequently referred for specialized treatment. Whether normal or pathological, dissociative states around the world display remarkable similarities and differences in phenomenology, distribution in the population, and local meanings that are amenable to empirical scrutiny. Abnormal states also show correspondences and variances in epidemiology, precipitants, psychiatric evaluations, treatments, and outcomes.

[1]The anthropological database on dissociative states is vast but focuses generally on the social context and the public performance aspects of these conditions rather than on the subjective experience of the affected individual, its psychiatric correlates, or neuropsychological substrates. This chapter discusses selective elements of two indigenous dissociative syndromes and does not pretend to cover exhaustively the broad field of cross-cultural dissociation.

These patterns of observable similarities and differences among dissociative states can be examined against the background of the sociocultural characteristics of the particular societies in which these states arise. Following this method, anthropologists and cross-cultural clinicians have generated multiple hypotheses and research questions regarding the relationship between culture and dissociation. Some of these are,

1. Is there actual epidemiological evidence of higher rates of dissociation in developing societies than in industrialized and postindustrialized nations, as would appear from the ethnographic record?
2. Does the field of dissociative forms in non-Western cultures narrow in proportion to increasing collective adherence to Western ideas of modernity and education?
3. Why do complex societies (e.g., those with a large population, social stratification, sedentary settlement patterns, dependence on agriculture) display predominantly one form of dissociative state—possession trance—whereas societies of lesser complexity (e.g., those with a small population, lack of stratification, dependence on nomadic hunting, gathering, and fishing) display another—trance without possession ideology (Bourguignon 1978)?
4. Why does the degree of these correlations also vary by geographical region (Bourguignon 1973)?
5. Why do certain regions throw forth a broad range of distinct culturally authorized dissociative states (e.g., South Asia), whereas others appear to produce only a limited number of forms (e.g., Northern Europe)?
6. Why do many members of certain societies (e.g., India) experience dissociation frequently as normal, whereas many members of other societies (e.g., United States) tend to characterize their dissociative states as pathological?
7. Why are certain dissociative conditions essentially restricted to men (e.g., *amok*; Schmidt et al. 1977), others markedly predominant among women (e.g., DID; Putnam 1989), and still others usually more prevalent among women but subject to variation by precipitating context and possibly by location or historical period (e.g., possession syndrome [Freed and Freed 1990a, 1990b] or *ataque de nervios* [Guarnaccia et al. 1993; Rubio et al. 1955])?
8. Why are some untreated dissociative illnesses chronic and unremitting (e.g., DID; Kluft 1985) and others episodic and relapsing (e.g., *ataque de nervios*; Guarnaccia et al. 1989a)?

126

9. Why do some involuntary dissociative states respond to symbolic treatment that is rapid and dramatic (e.g., exorcism), whereas others appear intractable to such healing procedures?

THE MEDICAL ANTHROPOLOGY PERSPECTIVE

How can these questions be addressed by empirical research? In light of this tremendous cross-cultural variation, what is the relationship between culture and dissociation? Specifically, how does culture interact with biology, environmental stressors, and individual psychology in the configuration of diverse pathological dissociative syndromes?

This chapter argues that a medical anthropology approach centered on the interpretation of meaning is essential for the investigation of these questions (Good and Delvecchio Good 1981). Such an approach would discover the networks of experiences, words, and interpretations that, "running together" in a given culture, give rise to particular illness forms (in our case, pathological dissociative syndromes). From the anthropological perspective, it is these *meaning networks* that play the biggest determining role cross-culturally in the configuration and distribution of illness and the nature of its sequelae. A *meaning network*—called *semantic* because it reveals the power of interpretation in shaping reality—includes "personal trauma, life stresses, fears and expectations about the illness . . . the metaphors associated with a disease, the ethnomedical theories, the basic values and conceptual forms, and the care patterns that shape the experience of the illness and the social reactions to the sufferer in a given society" (Good and Delvecchio Good 1982, p. 148).

Subjects neither invent syndromes anew nor express universal symptoms unmediated by culture; being *encultured* in the meaning networks of certain dissociative syndromes, they experience these illnesses naturally when their personal attributes, collective affiliations, and circumstances of suffering intersect with the semantic linkages of the syndromes. Thus the closer the characteristics of the encultured subject match the items in one of these networks, the greater will be the collective and individual (conscious and unconscious) pressure to express the corresponding syndrome.

In addition, within each culture, two other semantic factors influence the experience of particular forms of illness: their specific connotations of morality (i.e., their associations of *goodness* and *badness)* and their ability to function as vehicles of communication for distinct community messages (e.g., resistance against oppression, public resignation, group solidarity, reinforcement of tradition in the face of the incursions of modernity). Indeed, in situations in which certain social voices are actively muffled (e.g., women, the poor, the demoralized), these *idioms of distress* (Nichter 1981) may represent one of the main remaining powerful mechanisms of communication and redress. For more information, refer to the work of I. M. Lewis (1989), Janice Boddy (1989), and James C. Scott (1985).

Finally, these meaning networks, being cultural constructions, would be expected to show historical variation and to be significantly affected by drastic sociocultural dislocations, such as migrations (with subsequent exposure to new cultural mores) or changing sex roles. This historical mutability of meaning networks would help explain the significant variability over time of pathological dissociative states.

ATAQUE DE NERVIOS AND POSSESSION SYNDROME

This chapter illustrates the contribution of *semantic network* analysis toward cross-cultural research on dissociation by focusing on two indigenous conditions with marked dissociative features: *ataque de nervios* among Puerto Ricans and *possession syndrome* in India. The existing literature on the phenomenological, sociocultural, and psychological differences and similarities between these syndromes is discussed in light of semantic networks. Neurobiological data on these conditions are unfortunately not reviewed because they are currently unavailable. Throughout the text, multiple clinical and epidemiological correspondences and variances between the two conditions are first described and then correlated with known ethnographic differences and similarities between the two cultures. It is shown how the characteristics of the semantic networks of *ataque* and possession syndrome account for many features of these syndromes. In several places, there is question as to whether this relationship is not in fact *determinative* in that cultural factors appear powerful enough to direct and shape clinical and epidemiological realities. A constitutive role for culture in the patterning of illness states would not negate, however, the modulating activity of psychological, environmental, and neurobiological processes. Instead, cultural factors embedded in semantic networks would provide a mechanism that could account for a substantial portion of the great diversity and mutability of dissociative conditions introduced earlier and discussed in detail below.

INTRODUCTION

Ataque de Nervios

Case example. A 45-year-old Puerto Rican woman is suddenly confronted by the return of her estranged husband who, while intoxicated and in violation of a restraining order, is trying to break down her apartment door in order to take custody of their youngest child. While attempting to call the police, she notes the onset of an *ataque de nervios*. Her attentional focus has narrowed to the point where she is aware only of the numbers on the telephone dial. She is unable to complete the call, feeling that she is moving ineffectually and in slow motion. Her breathing becomes rapid and shallow, her heart rate accelerates, there is a feeling of heat rising from her chest to her head, and she begins to sob and scream uncontrollably. She runs back and forth to the door, starting to hit it and herself with her arms and fists, while her body undergoes generalized convulsive movements. Nevertheless, she is able to react to the frightened crying of her child, picking him up and taking him to a back room. After her husband leaves without being able to force his way into the apartment, she collapses to the ground, moaning softly. Some minutes later she gets up feeling exhausted, unsure whether she lost consciousness briefly, and remembering some details of the episode only sketchily.

Ataque de nervios ("attack of nerves") is a behavioral-experiential sequence indigenous to various Latin American cultures, including Puerto Rico, Dominican Republic, Cuba, and Central America. Among Puerto Ricans, it has received considerable attention in the psychiatric and anthropological literature for the past 30 years (Abad and Boyce 1979; Bird 1982; De la Cancela et al. 1986; Fernández-Marina 1961; Garrison 1977a; Grace 1959; Guarnaccia 1992; Guarnaccia et al. 1989a, 1989b, 1990, 1993; Harwood 1981b, 1987; Lewis-Fernández 1992a, 1992b; Lewis-Fernández and Kleinman 1994; Mehlman 1961; Rendón 1984; Rothenberg 1964; Rubio et al. 1955; Steinberg 1990; Teichner and Cadden 1981; Trautman 1961a, 1961b; Zayas 1989). Early research carried out during the 1950s and 1960s was hindered by methodological limitations that restrict its current usefulness. These limitations included sampling methods focused only on nongeneralizable subpopulations (i.e., military recruits and hospitalized suicidal migrants), the failure to distinguish whether the *ataque* label was ascribed to subjects by indigenous informants or by the researchers themselves, a lack of control subjects, and colonialist prejudice. This early work will be used in this chapter mainly as a window into the possible historical and cohort variations of the *ataque*. Sounder subsequent investigations combining psychiatric, epidemiological, and anthropological methodologies are just now becoming available and are locating the *ataque* in its sociocultural and psychiatric contexts and establishing its phenomenology and distribution.

Possession Syndrome

Case example. A 17-year-old Hindu woman is mending some clothing for her brothers-in-law under the close supervision of her mother-in-law 2 weeks after arriving as a new bride to the home of her husband's family in a different village, when one of her new in-laws makes fun of her sewing. The young woman puts her work down slowly, undergoes a general convulsion, rolls on the ground, and starts yelling loudly and incomprehensibly before losing consciousness. The family reacts by pinching her and attempting to wake her with other noxious stimuli. The young woman regains semiconsciousness with a start and a loud scream and identifies herself as the ghost of a dead cousin who committed suicide after her premarital sexual relations became public. The in-laws then threaten the spirit with other noxious measures for several minutes until the young woman again enters near-unconsciousness, moaning softly and breathing only with difficulty, signaling the temporary departure of the spirit. For a period of hours, she drifts between near-unconsciousness and full possession several times, then lapses into prolonged unconsciousness ending in sleep. After a brief period of disorientation upon awakening, she reports initially seeing the approach of the ghost but claims total amnesia for the subsequent events. Over the course of 3 weeks, these attacks of possession syndrome recur several times. During the episodes of full possession, the spirit demands from the in-laws more considerate treatment for the young woman. When provoked with pinching or hair-pulling, "she" becomes aggressive against the husband and his family by lashing out with fists and feet. The in-laws elicit the help of several exorcists who try harshly and unsuccessfully to expel the possessing spirit. Only after the young woman's father travels to see her in the company of another exorcist do her episodes of possession diminish. To pursue a cure, she leaves for an extended visit with her parents following up a referral to a regional healing temple.

Possession syndrome[2] is a behavioral-experiential sequence indigenous to several cultures of South Asia, including India and Sri Lanka. It shows substantial parallels with cognate instances of involuntary possession trance in an extremely diverse range of cultural settings all over the world. Descriptions of these possession trance illnesses are provided by Yap (1960) on Hong Kong, Kleinman (1980) on Taiwan, Eguchi (1991) on Japan, Ong (1987) on Malaysia, Stoller (1989) on Niger, Gussler (1973) on Southern Africa, Harwood (1987) on Puerto Rico, Pressel (1977) on Brazil, and Walker (1972) on Haiti. This chapter focuses exclusively on possession syndrome in India, where it has received considerable attention from anthropologists and psychiatrists for several decades (Adityanjee et al. 1989; Akhtar 1988; Carstairs and Kapur 1976; Castillo 1991; Chandrashekar 1981, 1989; Chandrashekar et al. 1980, 1982; Claus 1979; Freed and Freed 1964, 1990a, 1990b; Gold 1988; Harper 1963; Kakar 1982; Nichter 1981; Opler 1958; Pradeep 1977; Saxena and Prasad 1989; Sethi 1978; Shields 1987; Teja et al. 1970; Varma et al. 1970; Varma et al. 1981; Venkataramaiah et al. 1981; Wadley 1976; Ward 1980; Wig and Narang 1969). Despite this substantial effort, however, accurate assessment of several features of possession syndrome in India—particularly its phenomenology, epidemiology, and rates of associated psychopathology—is currently still problematic due to various methodological limitations of the available research. Most of the country—the second most populous in the world—has not been investigated; studies reviewed sometimes replaced indigenous categories with psychiatric diagnoses without reporting the former or did not distinguish episodes of voluntary possession from involuntary possession syndrome; most community-based reports were in the form of case series rather than systematic surveys (for notable exceptions, see Carstairs and Kapur 1976, Venkataramaiah et al. 1981); and extrapolation from research among psychiatric patients to global populations has proven inadequate due to the selective avoidance of psychiatric services by affected individuals who prefer indigenous treatments. This chapter reviews the current state of knowledge, pointing out gaps and discrepancies in the text.

Ataque and possession syndrome are comparable cultural categories that share some features in common with Western psychiatric syndromes:

---

[2] An umbrella term encompassing multiple names in Indian regional languages and dialects (Varma et al. 1970). Called *demonic possession* by Obeyesekere (1970) in his work on Sri Lanka.

They are normative conditions in their societies of origin, configured along descriptive parameters;[3] they are usually characterized as afflictions resulting from heightened stress; and they often result in distress, impairment, and increased use of health care resources. On the other hand, they also differ significantly from DSM or ICD diagnoses, which stand exclusively as representations of psychiatric pathology. *Ataque* and possession syndrome constitute broader idioms of expression, which may be used to convey totally normal emotions and cognitions and which connect with more comprehensive explanatory models for suffering, evoking moral and teleological dimensions and linking individual, collective, and even ecological contexts. In the case of India, possession syndrome may also communicate profound aspirations toward spiritual and psychological development (Claus 1979; Nichter 1981). In addition, the phenomenologies of these conditions are configured differently than those of Western psychiatric categories: Their prototypical presentations cut across DSM and ICD boundaries distinguishing thought, affective, anxiety, dissociative, and somatoform disorders (Good and Delvecchio Good 1982; Good and Kleinman 1985; Kleinman 1988; Lewis-Fernández 1992a; Weiss 1991; Wig 1983). Moreover, there is considerable variation among individual cases of *ataque* and possession syndrome in terms of Western boundaries. Although both conditions exhibit marked dissociative features, individual cases may additionally display diverse combinations of psychotic, anxiety, depressive, characterological, and somatic symptoms. The absence of diagnosable psychopathology in many subjects who have these syndromes and the psychiatric heterogeneity of the rest ensures that these indigenous conditions, as global categories, do not overlap with Western nosologies. Individual cases, however, may be amenable to psychiatric evaluation and treatment.

SEMANTIC NETWORKS OF ATAQUE AND POSSESSION SYNDROME

Indigenous views link *ataque de nervios* and possession syndrome, respectively, as cultural categories, to particular population groups (e.g., women),

---

[3]Organized as relatively invariant collections of symptoms rather than 1) etiologically, by attributed causation, or 2) according to ascribed treatment modality (see Good and Delvecchio Good 1982).

life circumstances, causations, treatments, and existential interpretations within each culture, forming stable and distinct semantic networks that nevertheless show historical variations.

Specifically, among Puerto Ricans, the semantic network of *ataque* currently includes women; middle age; rurality; urban poverty; *behavioral ethnicity*[4] (adherence to old ways) or, conversely, lack of modernity or formal education; and sudden inescapable suffering involving a person close to the subject, such as the death of a husband, child, or close relative. Linkage between *ataque* and noxious spiritual intrusion is more variable and tenuous. Some Puerto Rican *Espiritistas, Santeros,* and Pentecostals may attribute distinct spiritual causations to some *ataques,* but the semantic connections between those practices and the syndrome as a whole remain unclarified (Garrison 1977a; Guarnaccia et al. 1989a; Harwood 1981b; Lewis-Fernández and Kleinman 1994).

Among Indians, the semantic network of possession syndrome currently includes women; young adulthood; disadvantaged social status (low-to-mid caste); gradually worsening social and family stressors occurring in the absence of firm emotional support; *liminal* (boundary crossing) population groups and transitional life phases; and a "porous" self, spiritually vulnerable to the influence of gods/goddesses, spirits, and witches, and sensitive to ritual therapy.[5] Rurality and behavioral ethnicity—or lack of modernity and formal education—are also probably linked, but the research reviewed on this point is inconclusive (Castillo 1991; Claus 1979; Freed and Freed 1964; Kakar 1982; Nichter 1981).

Although they are linked to different regionally specific semantic networks, and thus culturally and phenomenologically distinct, *ataque* and

---

[4]For a discussion of *behavioral ethnicity,* see Harwood (1981a, p. 4). The term refers to a pattern of active behavior closely determined by "distinctive values, beliefs, behavioral norms, and languages or distinctive dialects" originating from the tradition of a particular ethnic group and acquired during socialization, which significantly shape the attitudes, social interactions, and institutional contacts (including health beliefs and practices) of the individuals who are socialized in them.

[5]Spiritual vulnerability may derive from the jealous actions of a witch; the attachment of a spirit; relational proximity to a family member, ancestor, or acquaintance who died under certain conditions of distress; and the crossing of geographical thresholds with symbolic connotations (e.g., stream, cremation grounds; Chandrashekar 1981, 1989; Chandrashekar et al. 1980; Claus 1979; Freed and Freed 1964, 1990a, 1990b; Opler 1958; Shields 1987; Teja et al. 1970; Varma et al. 1970).

possession syndrome appear to share at least one function in common: They embody and convey, in dissociative form, distress arising from feelings of loss, grief, anger, fear, and vulnerability precipitated by stressful experiences in the absence of firm emotional support. They appear as socioculturally cognate, but distinct, dissociative phenomena, making them appropriate research topics for a cross-cultural comparison of the interaction between the cultural construction and the brain-mind mechanism(s) of dissociation.

Phenomenology

Acute Episode

Episodes of *ataque de nervios* and possession syndrome show remarkable similarities and differences in their phenomenologies (Table 6–1). Both are precipitated by a broad range of stressful stimuli of diverse severities—from tense confrontations with relatives to instances of physical or sexual trauma—and result in a dramatic shift in consciousness, with associated semipurposeful acts (e.g., shaking, gyrating, falling to the ground) and occasional threatening gestures directed at self or at others. *Ataques,* however, 1) appear to display a more stereotyped onset (acute shift in consciousness characterized by a narrowing of attentional focus); 2) are typically triggered by sudden stimuli (e.g., news of the death of a close relative); 3) uniformly elicit an affective storm of primary subjective importance congruent with the stimulus (e.g., fear, grief, anger) and associated with somatic alterations (e.g., difficulty breathing, heart palpitations, dizziness, heat in chest); 4) rarely culminate during the attack in coherent vocalizations and demands; and 5) do not always result in loss of consciousness and partial or total amnesia for the event. Episodes of possession syndrome, on the other hand, 1) show considerable variation in onset, beginning at times as a nonspecific somatic prodrome preceding the identifying shift in consciousness; 2) occur most frequently in response to gradually intensifying stressors (e.g., incorporation of new bride into mother-in-law's home); 3) are less invariably associated with a primary affective storm with somatic alterations; 4) typically result during the altered state in coherent vocalizations and demands for assistance or improved treatment; and 5) are followed nearly always by transient loss of consciousness or marked disorientation and partial or total amnesia.

The main phenomenological difference between the two conditions,

134

nevertheless, lies in the realm of identity alteration. The substitution of the subject's identity by a culturally defined alternate personality, which is the primary characteristic of possession syndrome, is absent in *ataque,* as is any subsequent elaboration in the presence of the healer of the possessing identity(ies) and its relationship with the close contacts of the subject. This discrepancy may stem, in part, from differences in the semantic networks of the two syndromes with regard to conceptualizations of the self. Specifically, the Indian conception of the self appears to be more open to spiritual and human influence, more *porous* or *dividual* (see Castillo 1991; Shweder and Bourne 1984), than the equivalent Puerto Rican understanding. This

Table 6–1. A comparison of the clinical features of *ataque de nervios* and possession syndrome based on qualitative descriptions reported in the literature

Clinical feature	*Ataque de nervios*	Possession syndrome
Precipitating stimulus	Sudden	More gradual
Onset	Acute	Often subacute
	Stereotyped	Varied
Acute episode		
Shift in consciousness	+	+
Narrowing of attention	+	+/−
Affective and somatic disturbance	+	+/−
Semipurposeful actions	+	+
Aggressive gestures	+/−	+/−
Alternate identity	−	+
Coherent vocalizations	+/−	+
Visual/auditory hallucinations	−	+
Response to others	+	+
LOC or general unawareness	+/−	+
Partial or total amnesia	+/−	+
Exhaustion	+	+
Course		
Shifts of consciousness per typical episode	Single	Multiple
Duration		
Single shift	Minutes–hours	Minutes–hours
Total episode	Minutes–hours	Hours–weeks
Consecutive episodes	Weeks–years	Weeks–years
Relapse	Variable	Variable

Note. LOC = loss of consciousness; + = present; +/− = occasionally present; − = absent.

may comparatively facilitate the use in India of the supernatural language of possession to articulate the causation, dynamics, and therapeutics of distressing human relationships and circumstances. In addition, the discrepancy between the two syndromes may derive as well from a greater relative unavailability of alternate human social roles in the strictly hierarchical society of India (see Varma et al. 1981). The difference in this regard between Indians and Puerto Ricans may be relative, however, not absolute. This is suggested by the existence in Puerto Rico (apart from *ataque*) of several cognate conditions to possession syndrome, characterized by spontaneous involuntary possession of individuals by alternate selves regarded as different spiritual entities in *Espiritismo, Santería,* and the Pentecostal Church, and referred for specialized ritual treatment (Garrison 1977a; Goodman 1988; Harwood 1987; R. Lewis-Fernández, unpublished observations, 1985; Quiñones 1991; Sánchez 1978; Sandoval 1979). The cultural connection between these conditions and *ataque* remains unclear despite the seminal work of Harwood (1987) and Garrison (1977a, 1977b) on *Espiritismo.*

In India, permissible agents of possession vary by religion, region, and caste. The agents include spirits of deceased family members, in-law relations, known village acquaintances who died under specific conditions of distress, and minor supernatural figures of the Hindu pantheon (though involuntary possession by major deities is sometimes reported) and the Islamic spiritual world (Claus 1979; Freed and Freed 1964, 1990a, 1990b; Kakar 1982; Nichter 1981; Teja et al. 1970; Varma et al. 1981; Venkataramaiah et al. 1981). The agents tend not to include the personalities of alternate, living persons nor, apparently, simultaneous, ongoing possession by coconscious multiple personalities, as in DID, although consecutive possession by two or three agents is not rare. On occasion, a single agent may possess several members of a family over time or in succeeding generations (Freed and Freed 1990a, 1990b). The interpersonal transmission of possessing personalities suggests that the cultural reality of these social actors (the spirits) is more consensual and intersubjective in India than is the cultural reality of DID alters in the West.

Both *ataque* and possession syndrome permit a remarkable responsivity to environmental cues and the ministrations of others during the altered state despite frequent subsequent subjective reports of narrowing of attentional focus or general unawareness and loss of consciousness. Nevertheless, only subjects with possession syndrome occasionally describe after their attacks visual and auditory hallucinations of the alternate identity. Exhaustion is commonly reported after an episode of either syndrome.

Course

Syndrome courses show both similarities and differences. Although single shifts of consciousness in either condition usually last only minutes to hours, an *ataque* typically consists of only one such shift (ordinary consciousness–altered state–ordinary consciousness), whereas an episode of possession syndrome is frequently composed of many subsequent shifts of varying total duration that can alternate for days or weeks. This difference in episode morphology seems to correspond to the distinct nature of the precipitating stimulus for each syndrome (see the Precipitants section): *Ataques* tend to result from sudden stressors and are correspondingly brief, typically recurring only with subsequent exposure to sudden stimuli, whereas possession syndrome episodes usually emerge in the context of more prolonged, subacute stress. Perhaps because of this, the episode may take longer to resolve. Nevertheless, the course of both syndromes is single or episodic, not chronic and progressive, and return to premorbid functioning after attacks tends to be the rule rather than the exception.

Relapse

Rates of relapse of either syndrome are unknown. This is due in part to methodological issues, because nearly all of the studies reviewed were based on single evaluations focused on acute episodes or did not assess relapse rates. Anecdotal reports in the literature suggest a diversity of outcomes: Either syndrome may present only once (or as a brief series of successive episodes), recur only sporadically, usually in the context of heightened stress (e.g., an episode of possession syndrome after each of several pregnancies [Freed and Freed 1964]), or, alternatively, display a chronic pattern of recurring attacks that may be of variable duration (sometimes lasting years) and that may be markedly disabling (Abad and Boyce 1979; Freed and Freed 1964, 1990b; Guarnaccia et al. 1989a; Harwood 1987; Kakar 1982; Teja et al. 1970).

Epidemiology

As with phenomenology, comparison of epidemiological findings on *ataque* and possession syndrome reveals significant similarities and differences.

Prevalence

Prevalence rates for *ataque* among psychiatric cohorts have not been investigated systematically and thus cannot be compared with rates for possession syndrome among these populations (Tables 6–2 and 6–3). Rates for both syndromes among community-based samples, however, appear substantial, indicating that these conditions occur frequently in the countries in question, although methodological differences between the Indian and Puerto Rican research make precise comparison of rates difficult (e.g., eliciting period versus lifetime rates, interviewing index subjects versus informants, differential inclusion of children). In addition, there is evidence to suggest that the actual prevalence rate of possession syndrome is higher than indicated by the current systematic research, given anthropological reports of widespread occurrence (Claus 1979; Gold 1988; Harper 1963; Nichter 1981), cultural barriers to discussing the supernatural features of the syndrome with outsiders or in public (Freed and Freed 1990a), and the full caseloads of indigenous healers (Pradeep 1977). Preference for indigenous healers and avoidance of psychiatric services for treatment of possession syndrome (Carstairs and Kapur 1976; Chandrashekar 1989; Chandrashekar et al. 1980, 1982; Pradeep 1977) may account for the discrepancy in its reported prevalence rates between patient and community samples (Table 6–3).

The most significant difference between the prevalences of the two syndromes is the frequent epidemicity of possession syndrome—spread by a kind of psychic contagion in the context of known circumstances causing

Table 6–2. Prevalence of *ataque de nervios*

Type	*n* (total)	Rate (%)
Community survey: folk diagnoses		
All *ataques*	145 (912)[a]	16
Pathological *ataques*[b]	109 (912)[a]	12
Pathological *ataques*[b]	360,000 (3.5 million)[c]	10.4

Note. No data were available for clinician diagnoses of patient populations. Data are derived from a 1987 study using the Diagnostic Interview Schedule/Disaster Schedule (DIS/DS).
[a]Island population probability sample of ages 17–68.
[b]*Ataque de nervios* that met DIS severity criteria for a psychological symptom (consulting a physician or other professional, taking medications, or reporting some functional impairment) and could not be explained as resulting from physical illness or substance abuse.
[c]Statistical projection to island population probability (ages 17–68).
Source. Guarnaccia et al. 1993.

Table 6-3. Prevalence of possession syndrome

Type	Rate %	n/total	Duration	Study Sample	Methodology	Source
Patient populations: clinician diagnoses						
12-year period	0.93	400/42,877	1958–1969	Ranchi Mansik Arogyashala[a] total patients	Unspecified	Varma et al. 1970
7-year period	0.06	30/~50,000[b]	1973–1979	NIMHANS[c] total patients	Chart review	Chandrashekar et al. 1980
1-year period	0.2	6/2,651	1986	All-India Hospital[d] outpatients	Chart review	Saxena and Prasad 1989
Community surveys: folk diagnoses						
6-month period	0.97[e]	12/1,233[e]	1972	50% of village adults (age > 15) belonging to 3 castes	Symptom checklist	Carstairs and Kapur 1976
1-year period	3.5	41/1,158[f]	Unreported	Total population village school catchment area[g]	Systematic informant interviewing[h]	Venkataramaiah et al. 1981

[a]Psychiatric Hospital, Ranchi, Bihar.
[b]Approximation to number of total patients (unreported), based on reported number of possession syndrome cases and prevalence rate.
[c]National Institute for Mental Health and Neurosciences, Bangalore, Karnataka.
[d]Institute of Medical Sciences, New Delhi, Delhi.
[e]Includes only cases of "involuntary" possession.
[f]Excludes two cases of "voluntary" possession, or ~5% of all "cases."
[g]Near Sringeri, in West Karnataka (see Chandrashekar et al. 1982).
[h]Information gathered from one informant per family on all family members and village acquaintances.

subacutely elevated stress, such as local outbursts of measles—in contrast to the usually endemic pattern of *ataque* rates (Chandrashekar 1981, 1989; Chandrashekar et al. 1982; Freed and Freed 1990a; Varma et al. 1970; Venkataramaiah et al. 1981). However, two separate pieces of evidence suggest that the endemicity of *ataque* may be punctuated by intermittent temporary, but significant, elevations in *ataque* prevalence among specific cohorts in response to particular collective stressors, causing it to approximate at times the epidemicity of possession syndrome. First, early research documented high rates of *ataque*-like behavior (though without using the indigenous term) among two special Puerto Rican subpopulations recently exposed to cohort-specific stress: men inducted into the United States armed forces (Fernández-Marina 1961; Mehlman 1961; Rothenberg 1964; Rubio et al. 1955) and migrants to New York City—predominantly among young women (Trautman 1961a, 1961b). Among the latter, being hospitalized for an attack occurred most often within the first 2 years of arriving in New York. Presentations for admission decreased rapidly after that, suggesting a cohort effect of migration (Trautman 1961b).

Second, an anthropologically informed epidemiological survey in Puerto Rico recorded substantially elevated rates of *ataque* in the wake of a natural disaster, increasing in proportion to the degree of exposure among subjects (Guarnaccia et al. 1993). The Puerto Rico Psychiatric Epidemiology Research Project, directed by Dr. Glorisa Canino, performed the survey in 1987 on a probability sample ($N = 912$) of the entire population of Puerto Rico using a translated and culturally adapted version of the Diagnostic Interview Schedule/Disaster Schedule to which a question on *ataque de nervios* had been added (Bravo et al. 1991). The sample included a significant number of subjects affected by mud slides that caused substantial loss of life, destruction of property, and communal dislocation in 1985 (Canino et al. 1990). The rates of *ataque* were highest among subjects severely affected by the mud slides and intermediate among those moderately affected (Guarnaccia et al. 1993). These findings seem to indicate that *ataque* prevalence fluctuates according to exposure to both individual and collective stressors, following an endemic *and* a proto-epidemic pattern, and that the difference between it and possession syndrome in this regard may be one of degree rather than of kind.

Demographics

Sex. Both *ataque* and possession syndrome are more prevalent among women, but the degree of female preponderance in the research reviewed varied by syndrome, cohort, and selection methodology (Table 6–4). Nevertheless, all the community-based investigations of both syndromes and one psychiatric cohort study of possession syndrome reported women to men ratios of approximately 2–3:1. It should be noted, however, that some

Table 6–4. Prevalence of *ataque de nervios* and possession syndrome by sex

Subjects	Women (%)	Men (%)	Women: men	Sample	Source
Ataque de nervios					
Cases	20	10	2:1[**]	Community	Guarnaccia
Control subjects[a]	80	90	0.9:1		et al. 1993
Possession syndrome					
Cases	~3.5[b]	~0.08[b]	~44:1[***]	Clinical	Varma et al. 1970
Control subjects[c]	No data	No data	1:3		
Cases	~0.09[d]	~0.04[d]	~2:1[***]	Clinical	Chandrashekar
Control subjects[e]	No data	No data	1:1.4		et al. 1980
Cases	1.2	0.5	2.4:1[***]	Community	Carstairs and
Control subjects[f]	97	98	~1:1		Kapur 1976
Cases	5.4[g]	2[g]	2.7:1[**]	Community	Venkataramaiah
Control subjects[h]	94.6	98	~1:1		et al. 1981

[**]$P < 0.01$; [***]P unreported.

[a]Control subjects: community subjects without *ataques* ($n = 767$).

[b]Number of cases of possession syndrome divided by approximate number of men and women in total sample (derived from gender ratios reported for random sample of 14,399/42,877 total admissions).

[c]Control subjects: random sample of 14,399/42,877 total admissions, without exclusion of possession syndrome cases.

[d]Number of cases of possession syndrome divided by approximate number of men and women in total sample (derived from reported gender ratios for controls and approximate number of total subjects derived from reported number of cases and prevalence rate).

[e]Control subjects: total clinical sample (around 50,000, actual number unreported) excluding cases of possession syndrome. Gender ratio was reported globally for control subjects. $N = 50,000$ approximated from reported number of possession syndrome cases and prevalence rate.

[f]Control subjects: total community sample (1,233) excluding cases of possession syndrome (12) and subjects exhibiting voluntary possession (16 women and 6 men).

[g]Numbers confounded slightly by inclusion of two cases of voluntary possession (5% of total) on whom demographic information was not reported separately.

[h]Control subjects: total population of village school catchment area (1,158), excluding cases of possession syndrome (41) and subjects exhibiting voluntary possession (2).

Indian studies lacked the statistical analysis to establish significance.[6]

Sex distribution is not fixed universally, however. It may vary historically, according to evolving cultural sex attributions (Claus 1979; Nichter 1981), or in response to sex-specific stimuli. Evidence for the latter may be found in the high rates of *ataque*-like behavior reported among Puerto Rican men after military induction (Fernández-Marina 1961; Mehlman 1961; Rothenberg 1964; Rubio et al. 1955). Moreover, Indian villages may show geographic or, possibly, idiosyncratic variation. Freed and Freed (1990a) provided data on an Indian village where the unweighted proportion of women to men among cases of possession syndrome was 1.2:1 (women, $n = 21$; men, $n = 17$).

At present, the semantic networks of both *ataque* and possession syndrome link syndrome expression generally with women, attributing this connection to greater emotional and spiritual sensitivity among women (Lewis-Fernández and Kleinman 1994; Nichter 1981).

Age. The most robust difference in the demographics of the syndromes lies in their age distribution. In the more recent studies, *ataque* is significantly more prevalent among women over 45 years of age, whereas possession syndrome arises significantly more commonly among women under age 30 and especially among adolescents (Table 6–5). This difference may be taken to reflect distinct life-cycle distributions of stress among the two population groups. According to this explanation, Indian subjects would experience the greatest stress during adolescence and early adulthood and Puerto Rican subjects during middle age and later years. However, evidence of the great stigmatization of widows in India, regardless of age but occurring mostly in mature age groups (Castillo 1991; Harper 1969; Varma et al. 1970), and of the significant stressors experienced by Puerto Rican teenagers and young adults (Bourgois, in press; Harwood 1981b; Rodríguez 1991) argues against any simple age-linked hierarchical categorization of stressful experiences per se in these societies. It is more likely that the differences in age distribution of the syndromes stem from age-specific cultural attribu-

[6]The extraordinary disproportion of women to men among psychiatric patients reported by Varma et al. (1970) may represent selective avoidance of mental hospitals by men with possession syndrome or may represent bias because it was not reproduced among the psychiatric patients studied by Chandrashekar et al. (1980) nor among community subjects.

tions—part of each syndrome's semantic network—that mediate stress differently across the Indian and Puerto Rican age cohorts and determine the way it is experienced and coped with, including the relative appropriateness of discharging it through episodes of *ataque* or possession syndrome. These meaning networks, being cultural constructions, show historical variation and are significantly affected by drastic sociocultural dislocations such as migration. Similarly, we find what appears to have been a significant shift away from middle-age and toward adolescent prevalence—and perhaps toward greater suicidality—in the age distribution of *ataque*-like behavior among Puerto Rican migrants to New York City in the 1950s and 1960s. This shift probably reflects the impact of new age-specific stress response patterns on the migrants' cultural repertoire (Trautman 1961a, 1961b). A shift of this magnitude in the age distribution of an illness syndrome immediately following a pervasive cultural change such as migration may be explained

Table 6–5. Prevalence of *ataque de nervios* and possession syndrome by age

Subjects	Early adolescence	Mid-adolescence to early 20s	Mid-20s to mid-30s	Mid-30s to mid-40s	Over 45	Sample	Source
			Ataque de nervios				
Cases	a	15	←—42—→	43[**]		Community	Guarnaccia et al. 1993
Control subjects	a	25	←—45—→	30			
			Possession syndrome				
Cases	2.5	18	63.5	15.5	0.5[***]	Clinical	Varma et al. 1970
Control subjects	No data	No data	No data	No data	No data		
Cases	13	40	27	20	—[**]	Clinical	Chandrashekar et al. 1980
Control subjects	3	34	33	30	—[**]		
Cases	51	28	←—— 21[*] ——→			Community	Venkataramaiah et al. 1981
Control subjects	34	27	←—— 39 ——→				

[*]$P < 0.05$; [**]$P < 0.01$; [***]P unreported.
Note. Numbers indicate the percentage of subjects in each age group by case status.
[a]Only subjects over 17 included in study.

most parsimoniously by an alteration in the cultural associations relating to age embedded in the syndrome's semantic network.

Social factors. To date, correlations of both syndromes with several sociodemographic variables show considerable surface similarity. Individuals experiencing either *ataque* or possession syndrome are more likely to have received only limited formal education (Table 6–6); to belong to a disadvantaged socioeconomic group (mid-to-low caste in India, unemployed or out of the labor force in Puerto Rico; Table 6–7); and to be widowed, separated, or divorced (Table 6–8). These findings suggest a positive association between high social stress and vulnerability and the prevalence of both syndromes.

This association, however, is complex, because both the interpretation of experiences as stressful and the use of the syndromes as distress-reducing mechanisms are in large part culturally mediated (according to semantic networks). Illustrating this complexity is the finding that *ataque* and possession syndrome are not exclusively recourses of the most disadvantaged

Table 6–6. Prevalence of *ataque de nervios* and possession syndrome by education

| | Ataque de nervios | | | |
Subjects	< High school	High school +	Sample	Source
Cases	66	34[**]	Community	Guarnaccia et al.
Control subjects	49	51		1993

| | Possession syndrome | | | | | |
Subjects	Illiterate	< 5 years	5–10 years	10 + years	Sample	Source
Cases	45	37	18	—[***]	Clinical	Varma et al.
Control subjects	42	20	17	21		1970
Cases[a]	21	18	61	—[**]	Commu-	Venkataramaiah
Control subjects[a]	30	25	39	6	nity	et al. 1981

[**]$P < 0.01$; [***]P unreported.
Note. Numbers indicate the percentage of subjects at each educational level by case status.
[a]Includes only subjects 10 years old and over.

144

Table 6–7. Prevalence of *ataque de nervios* by employment status and of possession syndrome by caste and income

Subjects	Out of labor force	Unemployed	Employed	Sample	Source
		Ataque de nervios			
Cases	63	18	19[*]	Community	Guarnaccia et al.
Control subjects	51	18	29		1993

Subjects	High	Middle		Low	Sample	Source
		Possession syndrome				
		Caste				
Cases[a]	16[b]	46[c]		38[d†]	Clinical	Varma et al. 1970
Control subjects[e]	40	41		19		
Cases	33[f]	9[g]	58[h]	—[†]	Community	Carstairs and
Control subjects	37	16	47			Kapur 1976
Cases	17.5[i]	65[j]		17.5[k**]	Community	Venkataramaiah
Control subjects	36	31		29		et al. 1981

Subjects	Above Average[l]	Average[m]	Poor[n]	Sample	Source
	Income				
Cases	5[***]	73	23	Community	Venkataramaiah
Control subjects	6	71	23		et al. 1981

[*]$P < 0.05$; [**]$P < 0.01$; [***]P not significant; [†]P unreported.

Note. Numbers indicate the percentage of subjects in each social group by case status.

[a]Adjusted percentage for Hindu sample only.

[b]Brahmin, Bania, and Kayasthya castes. Mainly priests, businessmen, or their relatives.

[c]Goala, Teli, Rajput, and Bhumihar castes. Mainly landlords and oil pressers.

[d]Koeri, Kurmi, and Scheduled castes. Mainly poor agriculturalists and untouchables.

[e]Caste distribution for unspecified general patient sample at same Hospital reported by Rao (1966) and quoted in Varma et al. 1970.

[f]Brahmin caste. Mainly landowners.

[g]Bant caste. Mainly middle-level agriculturalists.

[h]Moger caste. Mainly fisherpeople.

[i]Brahmin caste. Mainly priests, businessmen, or landowners.

[j]Vokaliga caste. Mainly middle-level agriculturalists and service occupations (bakers, cart drivers).

[k]Scheduled caste/Scheduled tribe. Mainly untouchables.

[l]Above average: "income more than sufficient to maintain family."

[m]Average: "income sufficient to maintain family."

[n]Poor: "income not sufficient to maintain family."

in each society. Possession syndrome, for example, may be more prevalent among Indians with a few years of schooling than among the totally uneducated (Table 6–6), and its association with formerly married subjects may vary or apply only to psychiatric inpatients (Table 6–8). Among Puerto Ricans, anecdotal evidence suggests *ataque* may correlate more closely with indices of behavioral ethnicity than income or education. In addition, possession syndrome prevalence shows a complicated relationship with social caste among Hindu subjects (Table 6–7). First, cases are not infrequent among highly advantaged castes, such as Brahmins (see also Claus 1979; Freed and Freed 1964, 1990a; Harper 1963; Nichter 1981). Second, prevalence may correlate significantly with caste and not with income. Third, caste-specific rates may be lower among the untouchables (the most disadvantaged) than among castes in the lower middle of the social hierarchy. Finally, these rates show substantial historical variation (Claus 1979; Freed and Freed 1964, 1990a, 1990b; Nichter 1981). Castes are very complex social structures, organized along multiple cultural parameters (including myths, kinship patterns, race, vocations, literacy, diet, and religious ritual obligations), that affect every activity of daily life and interaction. It is not sufficient to reduce the impact of this cultural meaning system (operationalized as the semantic network) on the distribution of an indigenous syndrome to a decontextualized (and universalist) conception of *stress*.

Table 6–8. Prevalence of *ataque de nervios* and possession syndrome by marital status

Subjects	Never married	Married	Separated/ widowed/ divorced	Sample	Source
Ataque de nervios					
Cases	24	46	30[**]	Community	Guarnaccia et al.
Control subjects	33	49	18		1993
Possession syndrome					
Cases	3	75	22[†]	Clinical	Varma et al. 1970
Control subjects	18	79	3		
Cases	47	50	3[***]	Clinical	Chandrashekar
Control subjects	37	58	5		et al. 1980

[**]$P < 0.01$; [***]P not significant; [†]P unreported.

Note. Numbers indicate the percentage of subjects in each marital state by case status.

At present, the paucity of data on the cultural mediation of *ataque* and possession syndrome by various sociodemographic factors—including caste and class, race, behavioral ethnicity, religion, sexual orientation, and regional meaning systems—limits comparison of the syndromes on these variables to the surface similarities mentioned at the outset.

Rural/urban. The distributions of *ataque de nervios* and of possession syndrome by rural or urban area of residence cannot be compared on the basis of the research reviewed, given the tremendous geopolitical differences in this regard between the two countries and the paucity of data. Puerto Rico is small and highly urbanized, displaying subtle graduations of population density, making a rural-urban split problematic; whereas India shows dramatic contrasts between rural and urban settings, which yet remain essentially unstudied with regard to the distribution of possession syndrome.

Precipitants

Both *ataque* and possession syndrome are triggered by environmental, usually interpersonally grounded, stressful experiences eliciting strong feelings of loss, grief, anger, fear, and vulnerability. However, specific precipitants tend to cluster distinctly for each syndrome. *Ataque* is usually precipitated by sudden, often unexpected, distressing events involving persons close to the subject. Possession syndrome, on the other hand, typically arises during gradually worsening stressors of subacute duration involving persisting social or family conflicts or painful life transitions. Although this dichotomy is not absolute, it tends to hold for most cases. The precipitants most commonly reported by *ataque* subjects in the Puerto Rican epidemiological study are acute: an argument with a spouse or other close relatives, drunken behavior of a family member, an accident that threatened the life of a person close to the subject, death of a close family member, natural disaster (e.g., the mud slides in 1985), or the passing of a fright *(susto)* through a person (Guarnaccia et al. 1993). In contrast, typical precipitants encountered in the literature on possession syndrome are more gradual: incorporation of a new bride into the mother-in-law's home; delay in arranging marriage or in consummating it; forced marriage; widowhood; postpartum status; loss of family social standing; marital conflict, abuse, and neglect, at times associated with alcoholism; difficulty finding employment and financial difficulties; alienation from family support; and subordination to other family members and in-laws (Chandrashekar 1989; Chandrashekar et al. 1980; Freed and Freed 1964, 1990a, 1990b; Gold 1988; Harper 1963; Kakar 1982; Nichter 1981; Opler 1958; Shields 1987; Teja et al. 1970; Varma et al. 1970). In two studies, precipitants of this kind were identified directly in 11 of 15 (Teja et al. 1970) and 20 of 30 (Chandrashekar et al. 1980) subjects recruited from mental health settings.

Severity of the precipitants for *ataque* and possession syndrome ranges from mild-moderate to extreme. Although exposure to trauma during or after childhood has not been ascertained systematically as a risk factor, many of the precipitants discussed in the literature on both Indians and Puerto Ricans are obviously traumatic. For *ataque,* these include natural disaster, physical or sexual abuse, and sudden bereavement (Guarnaccia et al. 1989a, 1993). For possession syndrome, these include death of children, murder of husband, sexual abuse of a close friend, measles epidemic, physical abuse, and revelation of husband's incest with daughter (Freed and Freed 1964, 1990b; Gold 1988; Opler 1958; Teja et al. 1970; Varma et al. 1970).

In these cases, the authors seem to imply that the severity of the stressor itself is sufficient to cause the emergence of the syndrome as a defensive maneuver, and no further intrinsic psychic or social vulnerability in the subject is invoked. Alternatively, when either condition results from precipitants of milder severity, clinical investigators postulate the presence of factors exacerbating the vulnerability of the subject, such as hysterical, histrionic, and immature ego defenses (see the following Psychiatric Evaluations section) or underlying subacute/chronic interpersonal or sociocultural conflicts. Examples of the latter include marital argument or abuse, migration, poverty, discrimination, violence against women, precarious employment/source of income, childhood abuse or neglect, or family discord (Abad and Boyce 1979; Adityanjee et al. 1989; Castillo 1991; De la Cancela et al. 1986; Freed and Freed 1964, 1990a, 1990b; Guarnaccia 1989a; Harper 1963; R. Lewis-Fernández, unpublished observations, 1989; Opler 1958; Rothenberg 1964; Trautman 1961a, 1961b).

Anthropological analysis sees the existence of another kind of *vulnerability factor* in the role of the semantic networks, that is, in the traditional linkage of certain stressful life experiences to each syndrome in a cultural meaning network. These linkages tend to predispose individuals undergoing these experiences to express the corresponding syndrome as a mechanism for stress reduction and social communication. Possession syndrome, for example, appears to be linked to collective social experiences considered open to spiritual intrusion because of their transitional, boundary-crossing *(liminal)* nature, such as the regular crossing of village geographical borders (e.g., castes who gather forest products) and transitional life phases (i.e., birth, menarche, marriage, pregnancy, widowhood, and death; Claus 1979; Harper 1963; Nichter 1981). Participation in these social experiences will therefore act as a precipitant for possession syndrome in the now culturally vulnerable individual. The effect of semantic networks, traumatic exposures, character attributes, and social/interpersonal conflicts may obviously interact, modulating the expression (or nonexpression) of each syndrome within a given cultural range of clinical forms.

Psychiatric Evaluations

Most psychiatrists reviewed who investigated *ataque* or possession syndrome consider these conditions to be dissociative due to their appearance as shifts in consciousness occurring in the context of stressful stimuli, leading to an altered state resembling trance that is associated with apparently ego-dystonic and uncontrolled behaviors (along with perceptual changes and identity alteration in possession syndrome) and that is frequently followed by reported loss of consciousness and memory for the acute events. However, researchers disagree over the psychic origins of the dissociative processes and the normality of the underlying personality characteristics of the subjects. They also present differing data on the correlation of each of these syndromes with major psychiatric diagnoses.

Many investigators attribute the syndromes to intrapsychic hysterical, histrionic, or immature personality structures that predispose affected subjects to the return, in dissociated form, of repressed aggressive and sexual drives (see Fernández-Marina 1961; Mehlman 1961; Rothenberg 1964; Rubio et al. 1955; Trautman 1961a, 1961b on *ataque* and Kakar 1982; Teja et al. 1970; Varma et al. 1970 on possession syndrome). Other clinicians focusing on possession syndrome dispute this global pathologization of their subjects' character. They distinguish between the overall normal personality of the subject and specific hysterical intrapsychic processes that mediate the acute behavioral-experiential sequence of the syndromes (Chandrashekar 1981; Chandrashekar et al. 1980; Wig and Narang 1969). Still others, working separately in either syndrome, argue that some subjects' propensity toward involuntary dissociation may emerge from unassimilated traumatic childhood experiences that are sequestered in dissociated mental structures rather than from the pathological repression of inherent drives (Adityanjee et al. 1989; Castillo 1991; R. Lewis-Fernández, unpublished observations,

1989). These hypotheses have not been tested empirically.

Despite the prominence of their dissociative symptoms, subjects with *ataque* or possession syndrome seeking psychiatric care would be unlikely to fulfill criteria for any of the specified dissociative disorders in DSM-IV (American Psychiatric Association 1994). Several authors recently compared the nosological categories of possession syndrome and DID. They discovered major differences in presenting phenomenology, subjective experience, syndrome course, and response to treatment despite significant similarities in dissociative characteristics (Adityanjee et al. 1989; Castillo 1991; Saxena 1987; Saxena and Prasad 1989; Varma et al. 1981). Saxena and Prasad (1989) assessed the case records of 2,651 psychiatric outpatients in New Delhi and found 62 cases that fit into the dissociative disorders category of DSM-III. Over 90% of these did not qualify for the specified disorders and were diagnosed with atypical dissociative disorder, including six cases of possession syndrome. Assessment of the appropriateness of a dissociative disorder diagnosis for most *ataque* subjects is only now being performed (R. Lewis-Fernández, unpublished observations, 1989). However, clinical evaluations suggest most *ataques* with prominent dissociative features would currently also be assigned to the DSM-IV category of dissociative disorder not otherwise specified (González et al., in press).

Clinicians ascribing psychiatric diagnoses other than the DSM dissociative disorders to subjects with either *ataque* or possession syndrome find strong, though separate and distinct, correlations between each syndrome and different groupings of major mental illnesses (Table 6–9). Notably, the two studies with control subjects—Varma et al. (1970) in India and Guarnaccia et al. (1993) in Puerto Rico—serve to distinguish the psychopathological attributes of many syndrome subjects from relevant reference populations. In India, individuals expressing possession syndrome are more likely to be diagnosed with paranoid states or hysteria than their non-possessed, hospitalized counterparts and less likely to be assessed as having schizophrenia or manic-depressive illness, though they still received these diagnoses in substantial numbers. In Puerto Rico, *ataque* subjects are judged to be significantly more depressed and anxious than community respondents who denied the syndrome, earning diagnoses in these pathological categories much more frequently. They are also significantly more likely to experience self-destructive thoughts and suicide attempts, confirming similar early reports for subjects with *ataque*-like behaviors (Rubio et al. 1955; Trautman 1961a, 1961b). A similar association is also reported between suicidality and possession syndrome (Freed and Freed 1990b) but without systematic data. Unfortunately, significant methodological differences restrict comparison of these psychopathological correlates across the two syndromes. These include the study of hospitalized psychiatric patients with unspecified evaluation techniques by Varma et al. (1970) as opposed to the assessment of community subjects with a structured diagnostic ques-

Table 6–9. Results of psychiatric evaluations of subjects with *ataque de nervios* and possession syndrome and of control subjects

Psychiatric variables	Case subjects	Control subjects	Odds ratio[b]
Ataque de nervios[a]			
Depression	20	2	9.84
Suicidal thoughts	23	5	6.22
Suicidal attempt	21	3	8.08
Dysthymia	28	9	3.63
Generalized anxiety disorder	38	14	3.73
Panic disorder	9	0.4	25.08
Posttraumatic stress disorder	17	4	5.30
Alcoholism	16	14	1.15
Any affective diagnosis	30	12	6.18
Any anxiety diagnosis	40	12	4.02
Any DIS diagnosis	63	28	4.35
Possession syndrome[c,d,e]			
Schizophrenia	59	68	
Manic-depressive illness	11	24	
Paranoid states	20	0.25	
Hysteria	10	0.5	

Note. For the *ataque de nervios* group, numbers listed under case and control subjects indicate percentage of subjects meeting Diagnostic Interview Schedule criteria for that diagnosis. For the possession syndrome group, numbers listed under case and control subjects indicate percentage of subjects who received that diagnosis from hospital psychiatrists.
[a]The *ataque de nervios* section is reprinted with permission from Guarnaccia PJ, Canino G, Rubio-Stipec M, et al.: "The Prevalence of *Ataques de Nervios* in the Puerto Rico Disaster Study: The Role of Culture in Psychiatric Epidemiology." *Journal of Nervous and Mental Disease* 181:157–165, 1993. Copyright © Williams & Wilkins, 1993.
[b]The odds ratio reflects how much more likely it is that someone who reported an *ataque de nervios* met criteria for that diagnosis.
[c]From Varma et al. 1970.
[d]P values unreported.
[e]Percentages for other diagnoses unreported.

tionnaire by Guarnaccia et al. (1993). In addition, Varma et al. used unrestricted diagnostics, whereas Guarnaccia et al. assessed only certain DSM categories, excluding, among others, dissociative, psychotic, and personality disorders. Without further research, only juxtaposition of correlations is presently possible. Methodological differences probably also underlie the diagnostic inconsistencies found within syndromes between the controlled and uncontrolled studies reviewed. In addition to the absence of control subjects, the lack of clear structured diagnostic criteria regarding the category of hysteria in the studies of Rubio et al. (1955) and Teja et al. (1970) tend to bring into question their findings of disproportionate rates of hysterical character pathology among subjects with *ataque* and possession syndrome.

In summary, psychiatric evaluations of *ataque* and possession syndrome subjects in the literature reviewed usually describe the presence of some form of psychopathology. With *ataque,* this assessment is supported by subjects' own reports of poor health and use of popular and professional services for treatment of their *ataques* (Guarnaccia et al. 1993).

Clinical findings of high rates of pathology among subjects with *ataque* and possession syndrome run counter to traditional characterizations of both syndromes as appropriate expressions of normal experiences precipitated by suffering: strong emotions, in Puerto Rico, and examination of interpersonal dynamics in the language of supernatural relations, in India. Among the behaviorally ethnic of certain caste or class backgrounds, *ataque* and possession syndrome have been considered as *idioms of distress,* conveying without moral stigma social communications regarding resistance, a demand for group solidarity, and (at least in Puerto Rico) adherence to community traditions (De la Cancela et al. 1986; Lewis-Fernández 1992b; Nichter 1981). Indigenous idioms of mental illness, on the other hand, are usually heavily stigmatized in both Puerto Rico and India, conveying instead a sense of abnormality and social danger (see Delgado 1977; Garrison 1977a; Guarnaccia 1989a, 1989b; Harwood 1981b, 1987; Rogler and Hollingshead 1961 on Puerto Rico, and Carstairs and Kapur 1976; Chandrashekar et al. 1980; Davis et al. 1965; Khandelwal and Workneh 1986; Khanna et al. 1974 on India).

The discrepancy between psychiatric assessments of pathology and traditional connotations of normality may be the result of the following:

1. *Methodological artifact.* Appropriate expressions of distress via possession syndrome may have been overpathologized in the studies reviewed due to overinclusive diagnostics. Alternatively, the psycho-

pathology found in psychiatric inpatients with possession syndrome may be totally nongeneralizable to community samples reporting a similar behavioral syndrome. In Puerto Rico, it is possible that subjects experiencing *ataques* under culturally validated experiences of suffering systematically denied the syndrome to researchers inquiring about stigmatized psychiatric disorders, resulting in selection bias.

2. *Epidemiological shift.* The data on possession syndrome are too sparse to permit a historical perspective on epidemiological rates. But among Puerto Ricans it is possible that an shift in the epidemiology of *ataque* has occurred over the last decades in the direction of a disproportionately higher prevalence among psychopathological individuals, probably through the substantial reduction of culturally normal *ataques.*

3. *Cultural change.* Changing cultural attitudes toward the experience and expression of anxiety, depression, and, in some cases, psychosis may have resulted in a reinterpretation of both syndromes over time. Whereas these experiences in the past may have been considered aspects of normal life suffering, now only the most behaviorally ethnic may take this view. Instead, a growing number of Puerto Ricans and Indians may think of *ataques* and possession syndrome as abnormal, matching the psychiatric conception of psychopathology.

Treatment

Both *ataque* and possession syndrome are usually considered by the subject and his or her relations to require some form of assistance, but the decision to seek specialized treatment outside the family and the choices of therapy modality and caregiver appear to depend on two factors: the attributes of individual episodes and the behavioral ethnicity of the actors involved. In situations in either society in which all involved are behaviorally ethnic, simple cases occurring after normative precipitants and of brief duration might be treated with home-based remedies, group support, and collective attempts at relevant conflict-resolution. Referral to outside specialists would be reserved for refractory cases and complicated presentations or would be engaged in by recalcitrant family members in lieu of fulfilling expected problem-solving obligations. Alternatively, episodes of *ataque* arising in the midst of ongoing debate over the behavioral ethnicity of the relevant actors may receive early referral to either a single or multiple kinds of specialized caregivers (Garrison 1977a; Harwood 1981b; Lewis-Fernández 1992b).

As in the case of phenomenology, distinct spiritual conceptions appear to underlie the differences between Indian and Puerto Rican culture on the relative degrees of acceptance of biomedical versus spiritual diagnosis and therapy for each syndrome. Subjects with possession syndrome tend to prefer spiritual explanatory models and interventions and to avoid medico-psychiatric services (Carstairs and Kapur 1976; Chandrashekar 1989; Chandrashekar et al. 1980, 1982; Claus 1979; Gold 1988; Kakar 1982; Pradeep 1977), whereas *ataque* subjects in need of treatment seem to make more eclectic therapeutic choices, seeking the help of various medical, psychiatric, and spiritual caregivers, often all at once (Garrison 1977a, 1977b; Guarnaccia et al. 1989b, 1993; Harwood 1981b). The distinct character of these help-seeking patterns parallels the difference between the semantic networks of the two conditions: the network for possession syndrome contains a strong association with spiritual etiology, whereas this association appears more tenuous in the network for *ataque.*

When evaluated psychiatrically, *ataque* may be rediagnosed as panic disorder and treated with established psychopharmacological and behavioral modalities (Guarnaccia et al. 1989b, 1993). Possession syndrome and *ataques* conceptualized as spiritual afflictions may receive very similar treatments, including neutralization of the conflict or stress via the communal rituals involved in exorcism as well as the reformulation of the suffering into beneficent individual and communal practice via initiation into a spirit devotion cult—such as the Siri cult of South India or Puerto Rican *Espiritismo, Santería,* or Pentecostal Church (Claus 1979; Garrison 1977a; Nichter 1981; Harwood 1981b). In India, affected individuals may also be educated into the independent ritual roles of oracle (diviner), exorcist, or, rarely, *avatar* (*divine incarnation;* Castillo 1991; Claus 1979).

SUMMARY

This chapter reviewed the clinical, epidemiological, and anthropological similarities and differences between two indigenously defined conditions with marked dissociative features: *ataque de nervios* among Puerto Ricans and possession syndrome in India. In summary, these are as follows.

Similarities

Both syndromes stem from a dissociative reaction to a broad range (mild–traumatic) of stressors occurring in the absence of firm emotional support and leading to distressing experiences of loss, grief, anger, fear, and vulnerability. Phenomenologically, they share the following features: trance-like dissociations of consciousness, of sensorimotor control, and often also of memory (though this is less frequent in *ataque*), characterized by ego-dystonic acts and, occasionally, threatening gestures, which yet do not prevent marked responsivity to environmental cues. In both conditions, each dissociative shift lasts minutes to hours; exhaustion is typically reported immediately after an acute episode. Their course is variable, ranging from resolution after a single episode to years-long recurrence, distress, and impairment; however, it is typically relapsing, with return to premorbid functioning between episodes. Both syndromes are more prevalent among women and may present as an epidemic when a community is exposed to a collective stressor such as a natural disaster (though endemicity is the more usual pattern for *ataque*). The syndromes are more prevalent as well among more disadvantaged social groups, those with limited formal education, and the formerly married. In both conditions, there is debate whether they are due to hysteria or traumatically induced dissociation, and both syndromes are associated with suicidality. Also, they are often associated with diagnosable psychopathology and are seen indigenously as requiring care seeking, which may be home based. When referred to specialized spiritual healers, those who have these syndromes may receive similar treatments, including exorcism or admission into a trancing community. Anthropologically, both are associated with women, with marginalized social status, and with the social communication of resistance and a request for group solidarity but not with the expression of "mental illness," which is heavily stigmatized. Finally, both show substantial historical variation in sex and age prevalence and probably in the specific psychiatric diagnoses ascribed to each condition and in their indigenous assessment of normality or health.

Differences

Phenomenologically, the onset of an *ataque* tends to be more stereotyped (sudden shift in consciousness) than that of possession syndrome (variable somatoform prodrome to acute shift in consciousness). *Ataques* are characterized uniformly by an affective storm congruent with the precipitating stimulus and associated with somatic alterations, whereas the display of prominent affective and somatic changes in possession syndrome is more variable and depends on the subject's reaction to his or her interpersonal environment during an attack. Unlike *ataque,* possession syndrome displays dissociative identity alteration (possession trance) with marked culture-specific features, which is often associated with visual and auditory hallucinations of the possessing agent and with coherent vocalizations and demands during an attack. Loss of consciousness, disorientation, and partial or total amnesia after an acute episode is typical of possession syndrome and apparently less frequent or less severe in *ataque.* Acute episodes of *ataque* are typically composed of a single shift in consciousness, whereas those of possession syndrome are frequently composed of many subsequent shifts of varying duration that can alternate for days or weeks. Perhaps correspondingly, the former tend to be precipitated by sudden and discrete stressors, whereas the latter appear to result more often from gradually intensifying stress following their respective cultural associations. Despite the fact that the prevalence of both syndromes can display an epidemic pattern, *ataque* is primarily endemic, whereas possession syndrome is frequently epidemic. Currently, *ataque* is more prevalent among middle-aged subjects (over age 45), whereas possession syndrome is more prevalent among adolescents and young adults (under age 30). Psychiatrically, *ataques* are markedly associated with depressive and anxiety conditions, whereas possession syndrome subjects are more often given diagnoses of hysteria and paranoid states. (However, this discrepancy may be the result of methodological differences and/or local diagnostic practices rather than actual psychopathological differences.) Anthropologically, the Indian syndrome, and not the Puerto Rican one, appears to be linked to social groups that symbolize the traversing of boundaries (such as castes who regularly cross geographical village borders or persons undergoing transitional life phases [e.g., marriage]). Possession syndrome is also more closely associated with spiritual notions of causation (leading to the phenomenon of supernatural identity alteration) and, therefore, of treatment. *Ataques* usually present to multiple and diverse caregivers (including physicians), often at once, whereas subjects with possession syndrome tend to prefer spiritual healers and avoid professional services.

CONCLUSIONS

In this chapter, I have argued that, to a large extent, the correspondences and variances listed above among the features of these syndromes can be explained by parallel similarities and differences in cultural conceptions.

The characteristics of these syndromes are largely determined by cultural factors, and semantic networks coalescing indigenously around each syndrome constitute the direct mechanism for this mediation. The position advanced here is that sociocultural realities contribute at least as much to the phenomenology of experience—in this case dissociative illness—as psychological and neurobiological realities. *Ataque de nervios* may originate at least as much from the ideas and feelings about distress of the subject-cum-behaviorally ethnic Puerto Rican as from the subject-cum-traumatized ego or -cum-neurobiological entity.

This anthropological position may help explain certain features of *ataque* and possession syndrome noted in this chapter. First, some of the phenomenological differences between the syndromes could stem from the distinct configurations of their respective semantic networks, especially regarding differential cultural vulnerability to spiritual influence (and thus to the identity alteration of possession trance) and suddenness and duration of the precipitating stressors. Second, the lower prevalence of both conditions among men and persons with higher indices of socioeconomic status and modernity/education could reflect the absence of these human categories from both semantic networks. These syndromes are, in general, not available culturally to those social groups. However, some men who intersect the networks at other points (e.g., rurality, in Puerto Rico; disadvantaged caste, in India) would still have some access to them.

Third, the emergence of both conditions in certain individuals after nontraumatic precipitants could be the result of lower thresholds for syndrome expression in those persons who fulfilled network criteria. Fourth, the heterogeneity in course, relapse rate, and psychiatric status among subjects could derive in part from the attempted use of the language of the syndromes by individuals experiencing diverse mental illnesses with heavy biological loading. These persons may wish to evoke positive images of resistance and group solidarity and avoid the stigma and social powerlessness elicited by alternative cultural idioms of mental imbalance or weakness. Fifth, the more frequent predilection for local spiritual healers over psychiatric caregivers in the treatment of possession syndrome rather than of *ataque* may reflect the definite inclusion of spiritual elements in the Indian network and their more tenuous association in the Puerto Rican one.

Finally, the historical variations noted in sex and age distribution of *ataque*—and possibly in psychiatric correlates and local meanings—in response to changing stressors such as migration or military induction, and those in the caste valuations of possession syndrome, may derive from evolutions of the meaning networks over time in response to cultural developments. The biggest changes appear to stem from the effect of the ideology of modernity on these traditional idioms of distress. In time, the syndromes may exist only among the behaviorally ethnic, perhaps with alterations, or they may be supplanted altogether.

A cultural perspective is perhaps less challenging when advanced, as in this chapter, to explain cross-cultural events, which, viewed as "exotic" occurrences, seem to demand an explanation for their difference. It becomes more charged when it is applied to dissociative processes in general, therefore including those experienced in the West. Yet, obviously, the finding of significant constitutive effects of culture on dissociative phenomenology in one setting raises the possibility of a constitutive contribution of culture to dissociation in *any* setting. A cultural approach to Western dissociative syndromes (e.g., DID, depersonalization disorder, fugue) would argue that many of the features of these conditions are shaped by cultural factors organized in local semantic networks. Thus these conditions, just like *ataque* and possession syndrome, have their roots in particular interpretations of experience, not simply in biological or psychological mechanisms unmediated by culturally determined meaning systems.

Such a general cultural theory raises several challenges for overall psychiatric concepts of dissociation: First, this finding means that because cultures differ and dissociation displays different characteristics cross-culturally, *the dissociative disorder section in DSM needs to be expanded in order to include additional cross-cultural forms.* To be truly international, the DSM dissociative disorders section must contain a global sample of all dissociative conditions leading to distress and impairment. *Ataque* and possession syndrome have been shown to represent just such conditions, yet they do not fulfill criteria for any of the specified DSM-IV dissociative disorder diagnoses. DSM-IV improves this current nosological limitation a little through the inclusion of a new *dissociative trance and possession disorder* category in the appendix (Cardeña et al., in press; Lewis-Fernández 1992a). This is just the kind of expansion needed, but the fact that we are still recognizing "new" forms of dissociation should alert us to the possibility that key phenomenological features of the dissociative disorders worldwide still remain outside the DSM nosological system. The expansion of the professional nosology, therefore, is the first direct result of appreciating the role of culture in the configuration of illness states.

Second, the existence of cross-cultural diversity in dissociative syndromes may alter more than the diagnostic categories of the dissociative disorders. *Cross-cultural findings may support changes in the prevailing definition of dissociation itself.* Comparison of *ataque* and possession syndrome shows that, in the two cultures examined, discontinuities of sensorimotor control cluster with discontinuities of identity, memory, and consciousness as hallmarks of dissociation. Both syndromes are characterized by prominent repetitive movements and semipurposeful acts or complex (and often stereotyped) behaviors that are experienced as ego-alien and uncontrolled. These occur in conjunction with a trance-like state characterized by alterations of consciousness and memory and, in the case of possession syndrome, also of identity. Some instances of the syndromes are also associated with conversion-like phenomena, such as transient muteness or blindness.

This finding makes a difference because it argues for an expansion of the definition of dissociation in the DSM to include discontinuity of sensorimotor control among its cardinal features as follows: "a disruption in the usually integrated functions of consciousness, memory, identity, perception of the environment, *or sensorimotor control*" (the text before italic text is in DSM-IV, p. 477). This expanded definition would be closer to that of ICD, which already includes disorders characterized by psychogenic discontinuities of motor control and sensation (e.g., anesthesia) among the dissociative disorders.

One possible immediate nosological consequence of such a change for the DSM would be the reclassification of conversion disorder among the dissociative disorders. Another potentially more instrumental effect would be to direct research emphasis on the neurobiological mediation of dissociation to changes in the brain relationships between the primary and secondary motor areas and the rest of the cortex. Changes in control over these areas of the cortex at the onset and end of dissociative states may be easier to identify than equivalent changes affecting the extremely complex, disperse, and often harder-to-access brain structures mediating identity, consciousness, and memory.

Third, the constitutive role of culture in dissociative experience suggests that *the neurobiology and the psychology of dissociation may vary according to the cultural context in which they occur.* As described in this chapter, much of the particular phenomenology of a dissociative syndrome can be attributed to the patterning effect of culture on suffering. Culture may act as a reticulum of facilitations and inhibitions on the formation of experience, raising and lowering the thresholds (social, psychological, biological) for particular illness behaviors. Much as the presence or absence of a catalyst may determine the result of a biochemical process, the presence or absence of discrete cultural factors may determine the formation of a symptom. Whether the outcome of this (social or biochemical) process is or is not a sign of abnormality may depend on whether the process took place in the presence or the absence of the catalyst. Without the catalyst, the reaction might proceed only in the presence of nonhomeostatic, extraordinary forces and thus be a sign of pathology. With the catalyst, it might yield the product from nonpathological, homeostatic precursors and thus be an unremarkable occurrence. In this way, not only the mechanism itself (the physics and biochemistry of the process) but its meaning (normality or pathology) is affected by the context (the presence or absence of the catalyst). Neurobiologists and psychologists must, therefore, be prepared to contextualize their studies of dissociative mechanisms (the reaction) within specific cultural parameters (the catalyst) or face the risk of confounding their findings with the effects of differential cultural predispositions.

To take an example from this review: Despite multiple phenomenological similarities, the two syndromes reviewed are clearly different with regard to the dissociation of identity; it is present in possession syndrome and absent in *ataque*. The text suggests that cultural sources of this discrepancy may be found in the existence among possessed Indians (as compared to Puerto Ricans with *ataques)* of 1) greater porosity or permeability of the self and 2) more pervasive spiritual notions of causality. These factors may predispose affected Indians toward identity alteration as an embodied expression of suffering. Such a facilitated *(catalyzed)* identity alteration would probably be more transient (as is usually the case in possession syndrome) and constitute a sign of lesser pathology than a similar experience occurring in a person whose cultural context predisposes *against* sudden and marked changes in identity. In these more bounded and individualistic persons *(uncatalyzed),* greater psychological violence would be required in order to overcome the cultural barrier against dissociation of the self and produce identity alteration. Consequently, the resulting effect (a *shattered* self) would be more pathological and pervasive. This may be why, in the highly individualistic societies of North America, extreme trauma is required to produce DID, a disorder of chronic and severe identity alteration.

The existence of just this kind of differential cultural barrier to dissociation has recently been postulated, based in part, as is suggested here, on the cultural characteristics of the affected self (Martínez-Taboas 1991; Ross 1991). I would argue that this barrier can be quite symptom specific, based on the particular cultural characteristics that create the barrier in the first place. It can therefore block a given expression of dissociation (identity alteration) in one cultural syndrome (e.g., *ataque)* but not in another (possession syndrome) while permitting the appearance of other dissociative symptoms in either condition. The existence of such a barrier would mean that dissociative symptoms that appear on the surface to be phenomenologically similar may in fact have distinct psychological and neurobiological mechanisms. Alternatively, similar predisposing factors (e.g., trauma) may result either in different dissociative syndromes or in distinct psychiatric reactions altogether, according to the interaction of differently interpreted stressors, cultural barriers to dissociation, and configurations of syndromes determined by local semantic networks. Therefore, the cultural study of dissociation argues that neurobiological or psychological mechanisms associated with one dissociative illness in one culture cannot be generalized too broadly without empirical comparison to other dissociative syndromes in other cultures.

In conclusion, this chapter has argued for the inclusion of cultural studies as a fundamental partner in the course of scientific psychiatric research on dissociation. Dissociative illnesses are not the product of universal mechanistic abnormalities of neurobiology or psychology existing independently of cultural meaning. A serious look at the great diversity of dissociative states cross-culturally leads to an appreciation of the constitutive role of culture in this diversity. Consequently, this knowledge raises basic questions about 1) the completeness of DSM-IV nosology regarding dissociative disorders worldwide, 2) the adequacy of current definitions of dissociation that deemphasize discontinuities in sensorimotor control, and 3) the research assumption that studies on the neurobiological and psychological mechanisms of dissociation are universally applicable and *culture free.*

The fields of anthropology and psychiatry have suffered in the past from their division into two separate streams of knowledge (Kleinman 1988). The culture-mind-body investigation of dissociation would benefit greatly from their integration, offering further proof of the continuing need for the development of bridging research methodologies.

REFERENCES

Abad V, Boyce E: Issues in psychiatric evaluations of Puerto Ricans: a socio-cultural perspective. Journal of Operational Psychiatry 10:28–39, 1979

Adityanjee, Raju GSP, Khandelwal SK: Current status of multiple personality disorder in India. Am J Psychiatry 146:1607–1610, 1989

Akhtar S: Four culture-bound psychiatric syndromes in India. Int J Soc Psychiatry 34:70–74, 1988

American Psychatric Association: Diagnostic and Statistical Manual of Mental Disorders, 4th Edition. Washington, DC, American Psychiatric Association, 1994

Bird HR: The cultural dichotomy of colonial people. J Am Acad Psychoanal 10:195–209, 1982

Boddy J: Wombs and Alien Spirits: Women, Men, and the *Zâr* Cult in Northern Sudan. Madison, WI, University of Wisconsin Press, 1989

Bourgois P: From Jíbaro to crack dealer: confronting the restructuring of capitalism in Spanish Harlem, in Articulating Hidden Histories: Festschrift for Eric Wolf. Edited by Rapp R, Schneider J. Berkeley, University of California Press (in press)

Bourguignon E: Introduction: a framework for the comparative study of altered states of consciousness, in Religion, Altered States of Consciousness, and Social Change. Edited by Bourguignon E. Columbus, OH, Ohio State University Press, 1973, pp 3–35

Bourguignon E: Spirit possession and altered states of consciousness: the evolution of an inquiry, in The Making of Psychological Anthropology. Edited by Spindler GD. Berkeley, University of California Press, 1978, pp 479–515

Bravo M, Canino GJ, Rubio-Stipec M, et al: A cross-cultural adaptation of a psychiatric epidemiological instrument: the Diagnostic Interview Schedule's adaptation in Puerto Rico. Culture, Medicine, and Psychiatry 15:1–18, 1991

Brown S: The Heyday of Spiritualism. New York, Hawthorn, 1970

Canino G, Bravo M, Rubio-Stipec M, et al: The impact of disaster on mental health: prospective and retrospective analyses. International Journal of Mental Health 19:51–69, 1990

Cardeña E, Lewis-Fernández R, Bear D, et al: Dissociative disorders, in Sourcebook for DSM-IV. Edited by Frances AJ. Washington, DC, American Psychiatric Association Press (in press)

Carlson ET: The history of dissociation until 1880, in Split Minds/Split Brains: Historical and Current Perspectives. Edited by Quen JM. New York, New York University Press, 1986, pp 7–30

Carstairs GM, Kapur RL: The Great Universe of Kota: Social Change and Mental Disorder in an Indian Village. Berkeley, University of California Press, 1976

Castillo RJ: Culture, trance and mental Illness: divided consciousness in South Asia. Unpublished doctoral dissertation. Harvard University, January 1991

Chandrashekar CR: A victim of an epidemic of possession syndrome. Indian Journal of Psychiatry 23:370–372, 1981

Chandrashekar CR: Possession syndrome in India, in Altered States of Consciousness and Mental Health. Edited by Ward CA. Newbury Park, CA, Sage, 1989, pp 79–95

Chandrashekar CR, Channabasavanna SM, Venkataswamy RM: Hysterical possession syndrome. Indian Journal of Psychological Medicine 3:35–40, 1980

Chandrashekar CR, Venkataramaiah V, Mallikarjunaiah M, et al: An epidemic of possession in a school in South India. Indian Journal of Psychiatry 24:295–299, 1982

Claus PJ: Spirit possession and spirit mediumship from the perspective of Tulu oral traditions. Culture, Medicine, and Psychiatry 3:29–52, 1979

Davis RB, Gupta NC, Davis AB: The first ten years: some phenomena of a private psychiatric hospital. Indian Journal of Psychiatry 7:231–242, 1965

De la Cancela V, Guarnaccia PJ, Carrillo E: Psychosocial distress among Latinos: a critical analysis of ataques de nervios. Humanity and Society 10:431–447, 1986

Delgado M: Puerto Rican spiritualism and the social work profession. Social Casework, October 1977, pp 451–458

Eguchi S: Between folk concepts of illness and psychiatric diagnosis: *kitsune-tsuki* (fox possession) in a mountain village of Western Japan. Culture, Medicine, and Psychiatry 15:421–451, 1991

Ellenberger HF: The Discovery of the Unconscious: The History and Evolution of Dynamic Psychiatry. New York, Basic Books, 1970

Fernández-Marina R: The Puerto Rican syndrome: its dynamics and cultural determinants. Psychiatry 24:79–82, 1961

Freed SA, Freed RS: Spirit possession as illness in a North Indian village. Ethnology 3:152–171, 1964

Freed RS, Freed SA: Ghost illness in a North Indian village. Soc Sci Med 30:617–623, 1990a

Freed SA, Freed RS: Taraka's ghost: for a new bride in North India, stress takes many forms. Natural History 99:84–91, 1990b

Garrison V: The "Puerto Rican syndrome" in psychiatry and espiritismo, in Case Studies in Spirit Possession. Edited by Crapanzano V, Garrison V. New York, Wiley, 1977a, pp 383–449

Garrison V: Doctor, *espiritista* or psychiatrist? Health-seeking behavior in a Puerto Rican neighborhood of New York City. Med Anthropol 1:65–191, 1977b

Gold AG: Spirit possession perceived and performed in rural Rajasthan. Contributions to Indian Sociology 22:35–63, 1988

González C, Lewis-Fernández R, Griffith EE, et al: Cultural considerations regarding the dissociative disorders, in Sourcebook for DSM-IV. Edited by Frances AJ, Washington, DC, American Psychiatric Association Press (in press)

Good BJ, Delvecchio Good MJ: The meaning of symptoms: a cultural hermeneutic model for clinical practice, in The Relevance of Social Science for Medicine. Edited by Eisenberg L, Kleinman A. Dordrecht, Reidel, 1981, pp 165–196

Good BJ, Delvecchio Good MJ: Toward a meaning-centered analysis of popular illness categories: "fright-illness" and "heart distress" in Iran, in Cultural Conceptions of Mental Health and Therapy. Edited by Marsella AJ, White GM. Dordrecht, Reidel, 1982, pp 141–166

Good BJ, Kleinman A: Culture and anxiety: cross-cultural evidence for the patterning of anxiety disorders, in Anxiety and the Anxiety Disorders. Edited by Tuma H, Mazur J. New York, Erlbaum, 1985, pp 297–323

Goodman FD: How About Demons? Possession and Exorcism in the Modern World. Bloomington, IN, Indiana University Press, 1988

Grace WJ: Ataque. New York Medicine 15:12–13, 1959

Guarnaccia PJ: *Ataques de nervios* in Puerto Rico: culture-bound syndrome or popular illness? Med Anthropol 15:1–14, 1992

Guarnaccia PJ, De la Cancela V, Carrillo E: The multiple meaning of ataques de nervios in the Latino community. Med Anthropol 11:47–62, 1989a

Guarnaccia PJ, Rubio-Stipec M, Canino G: Ataques de nervios in the Puerto Rican Diagnostic Interview Schedule: the impact of cultural categories on psychiatric epidemiology. Culture, Medicine, and Psychiatry 13:275–295, 1989b

Guarnaccia PJ, Good BJ, Kleinman A: A critical review of epidemiological studies of Puerto Rican mental health. Am J Psychiatry 147:1449–1456, 1990

Guarnaccia PJ, Canino G, Rubio-Stipec M, et al: The Prevalence of *ataques de nervios* in the Puerto Rico Disaster Study: the role of culture in psychiatric epidemiology. J Nerv Ment Dis 181:159–167, 1993

Gurney E, Myers FWH, Podmore F: Phantasms of the Living. London, Kegan Paul, 1918

Gussler J: Social change, ecology, and spirit possession among the South African Nguni, in Religion, Altered States of Consciousness, and Social Change. Edited by Bourguignon E. Columbus, OH, Ohio State University Press, 1973, pp 88–126

Harper EB: Spirit possession and social structure, in Anthropology on the March: Recent Studies of Indian Beliefs, Attitudes and Social Institutions. Edited by Ratnam B. Madras, Madras Book Center, 1963, pp 165–177

Harper EB: Fear and the status of women. Southwestern Journal of Anthropology 25:81–95, 1969

Harwood A: Introduction, in Ethnicity and Medical Care. Edited by Harwood A. Cambridge, MA, Harvard University Press, 1981a, pp 1–36

Harwood A: Mainland Puerto Ricans, in Ethnicity and Medical Care. Edited by Harwood A. Cambridge, MA, Harvard University Press, 1981b, pp 397–481

Harwood A: RX: Spiritist as Needed. Ithaca, NY, Cornell University Press, 1987

James W: Essays in psychical research, Vol 16, in The Works of William James. Edited by Burkhardt FH, Bowers F. Cambridge, MA, Harvard University Press, 1986

Janet P: The Major Symptoms of Hysteria (1907). New York, Hafner, 1965

Kakar S: Shamans, Mystics, and Doctors. New York, Knopf, 1982

Khandelwal SK, Workneh F: Perceptions of mental illness by medical students. Indian Journal of Psychological Medicine 9:26–32, 1986

Khanna BC, Wig NN, Varma VK: General hospital psychiatric clinic: an epidemiological study. Indian Journal of Psychiatry 16:211–220, 1974

Kleinman A: Patients and Healers in the Context of Culture: An Exploration of the Borderland between Anthropology, Medicine, and Psychiatry. Berkeley, University of California Press, 1980

Kleinman A: Rethinking Psychiatry: From Cultural Category to Personal Experience. New York, Free Press, 1988

Kluft RP: The natural history of multiple personality disorder, in Childhood Antecedents of Multiple Personality. Edited by Kluft RP. Washington, DC, American Psychiatric Press, 1985, pp 197–238

Lewis IM: Ecstatic Religion: A Study of Shamanism and Spirit Possession. London, Routledge, 1989

Lewis-Fernández R: The proposed DSM-IV trance and possession disorder category: potential benefits and risks. Transcultural Psychiatric Research Review 29:301–317, 1992a

Lewis-Fernández R: *Ataques de nervios* or panic attacks: an embodied contestation of Puerto Rican ethnicity. Paper presented at the panel, Healing, Bodily Practices, and Caribbean Ethnicity, at the annual meeting of the American Anthropological Association, San Francisco, CA, 1992b

Lewis-Fernández R, Kleinman A: Culture, personality, and psychopathology. J Abnorm Psychol 103:67–71, 1994

Martínez-Taboas A: Multiple Personality Disorder as seen from a social constructionist viewpoint. Dissociation 4:129–133, 1991

Mehlman RD: The Puerto Rican syndrome. Am J Psychiatry 118:328–332, 1961

Nichter M: Idioms of distress: alternatives in the expression of psychosocial distress: a case study from South India. Culture, Medicine, and Psychiatry 5:379–408, 1981

Obeyesekere G: The idiom of demonic possession: a case study. Soc Sci Med 4:97–111, 1970

Ong A: Spirits of Resistance and Capitalist Discipline: Factory Women in Malaysia. Albany, NY, State University of New York Press, 1987

Opler ME: Spirit possession in a rural area of Northern India, in Reader in Comparative Religion: An Anthropological Approach. Edited by Lessa WA, Vogt EZ. Evanston, IL, Row, Peterson, 1958, pp 553–566

Pradeep D: A study of clientele and practice of a traditional healer. Unpublished doctoral dissertation, Bangalore University, India, 1977; Quoted in Chandrashekar CR: Possession syndrome in India, in Altered States of Consciousness and Mental Health: A Cross-Cultural Perspective. Edited by Ward CA. Newbury Park, CA, Sage, 1989, pp 79–95

Pressel E: Negative spirit possession in experienced Brazilian Umbanda spirit mediums, in Case Studies in Spirit Possession. Edited by Crapanzano V, Garrison V. New York, Wiley, 1977, pp 333–364

Putnam FW: Diagnosis and Treatment of Multiple Personality Disorder. New York, Guilford, 1989

Quiñones S: Exorcism: a therapeutic intervention, in Claves Psicológicas en Nuestra América: Visión Puertorriqueña. Edited by Nurse-Allende LI, Sumaya-Laborde I, Vásquez MA, et al. San Juan, PR, Libros Homines, 1991, pp 221–229

Rendón M: Myths and stereotypes in minority groups. Int J Soc Psychiatry 30:297–309, 1984

Rodríguez CE: Puerto Ricans, Born in the U.S.A. Boulder, CO, Westview, 1991

Rogler LH, Hollingshead AB: The Puerto Rican spiritualist as a psychiatrist. American Journal of Sociology 67:17–21, 1961

Ross CA: The dissociated executive self and the cultural dissociation barrier. Dissociation 4:55–61, 1991

Rothenberg A: Puerto Rico and aggression. Am J Psychiatry 120:962–970, 1964

Rubio M, Urdaneta M, Doyle JL: Psychopathologic reaction patterns in the Antilles Command. United States Armed Forces Medical Journal 6:1767–1772, 1955

Sánchez J: La Religión de los Orichas. Hato Rey, PR, Ramallo, 1978

Sandoval MC: Santería as a mental health care system: an historical overview. Soc Sci Med 13B:137–151, 1979

Saxena S: "Simple dissociative disorder": a subcategory in DSM-III-R (letter)? Am J Psychiatry 144:524–525, 1987

Saxena S, Prasad KVSR: DSM-III subclassification of dissociative disorders applied to psychiatric outpatients in India. Am J Psychiatry 146:261–262, 1989

Schmidt K, Hill L, Guthrie G: Running Amok. Int J Soc Psychiatry 23:264–274, 1977

Scott JC: Weapons of the Weak: Everyday Forms of Peasant Resistance. New Haven, CT, Yale University Press, 1985

Sethi BB: Culture bound syndromes in India. Indian Journal of Psychiatry 20:295–296, 1978

Shields NK: Healing spirits of South Kanara. Culture, Medicine, and Psychiatry 11:417–435, 1987

Shweder RA, Bourne EJ: Does the concept of the person vary cross-culturally? in Culture Theory: Essays on Mind, Self, and Emotion. Edited by Shweder RA, LeVine RA. Cambridge, MA, Cambridge University Press, 1984

Steinberg M: Transcultural issues in psychiatry: the ataque and multiple personality disorder. Dissociation 3:287–289, 1990

Stoller P: Fusion of the Worlds: An Ethnography of Possession among the Songhay of Niger. Chicago, IL, University of Chicago Press, 1989

Teichner VJ, Cadden JJ: The Puerto Rican patient: some historical, cultural and psychological aspects. J Am Acad Psychoanal 9:277–289, 1981

Teja JS, Khanna BS, Subrahmanyam TB: "Possession states" in Indian patients. Indian Journal of Psychiatry 12:71–87, 1970

Trautman EC: The suicidal fit: a psychobiological study of Puerto Rican immigrants. Arch Gen Psychiatry 5:76–83, 1961a

Trautman EC: Suicide attempts of Puerto Rican immigrants. Psychiatric Q 35:544–554, 1961b

Varma LP, Srivastava DK, Sahay RN: Possession syndrome. Indian Journal of Psychiatry 12:58–70, 1970

Varma VK, Bouri M, Wig NN: Multiple personality in India: comparison with hysterical possession state. Am J Psychother 35:113–120, 1981

Venkataramaiah V, Mallikarjunaiah M, Chandrashekar CR, et al: Possession syndrome: an epidemiological study in West Karnataka. Indian Journal of Psychiatry 23:213–218, 1981

Wadley SS: The spirit "rides" or the spirit "comes": possession in a North Indian village, in The Realm of the Extra-Human: Agents and Audiences. Edited by Bharati A. The Hague, Mouton, 1976, pp 233–251

Walker SS: Ceremonial Spirit Possession in Africa and Afro-America: Forms, Meanings, and Functional Significance for Individuals and Social Groups. Leiden, Brill, 1972

Ward C: Spirit possession and mental health: a psycho-anthropological perspective. Human Relations 33:149–163, 1980

Weiss MG: Culture and the diagnosis of somatoform and dissociative disorders: comments and considerations based on González and Griffith. Paper presented at the Cultural Issues and Psychiatric Diagnosis Conference, Pittsburgh, PA, April 11–12, 1991

Wig NN: DSM-III: A perspective from the Third World, in International Perspectives on DSM-III. Edited by Spitzer RL, Williams JBW, Skodol AE. Washington, DC, American Psychiatric Press, 1983, pp 79–89

Wig NN, Narang RL: Hysterical psychosis. Indian Journal of Psychiatry 11:93–100, 1969

Yap PM: The possession syndrome: a comparison of Hong Kong and French findings. The Journal of Mental Science 106:114–137, 1960

Zayas LH: A retrospective on "the suicidal fit" in mainland Puerto Ricans: research issues. Hispanic Journal of Behavioral Sciences 11:46–57, 1989

Section IV

Dissociation: Mind and Body

CHAPTER 7

Dissociation and Physical Illness

Colin A. Ross, M.D.

D issociation has been a topic of renewed scientific and clinical interest over the last decade (Putnam 1989; Ross 1989). Hilgard's (1977) neodissociation theory and studies by Ludwig et al. (1972) inaugurated contemporary scientific study of the topic. At the same time, pioneering clinical work on dissociative identity disorder (DID; formerly called multiple personality disorder) in the late 1970s culminated in the creation of a separate section for dissociative disorders in DSM-III in 1980 (American Psychiatric Association 1980). This event, combined with landmark articles published in the same year (Bliss 1980; Coons 1980; Greaves 1980; Rosenbaum 1980), set in motion an exponential increase in the rate of diagnosis of DID and publications on dissociation (Goettman et al. 1991) that has continued up to the present.

In the last few years, there has been increasing recognition of the work on dissociation done in the nineteenth and early twentieth centuries by Freud, Breuer, Janet, Charcot, Prince, Binet, and others (Ellenberger 1970; Putnam 1989; Ross 1989; van der Kolk and van der Hart 1989). For over half a century, dissociation fell into obscurity and this work was lost; one aspect of the recovery of this heritage has been recent interest in the psychophysiology of dissociation and the relationship between dissociation and physical illness (Alvarado 1989).

Clinicians working with dissociative patients are impressed by the wide range of somatic symptoms and phenomena they report, as summarized in three reviews of the relevant literature (Coons 1988; Loewenstein 1990; Putnam 1984). Despite a great deal of clinical interest in the subject, however, only a small amount of systematic research has focused on the psychophysiology of dissociation (Putnam 1991); therefore, our understanding remains preliminary and tentative.

In this chapter, I present an overview of conceptual issues concerning the relationship between dissociation and physical illness, briefly discuss the available measures of dissociation and somatization, and conclude by describing some of my own research in the area and by suggesting directions for future development of the field. Because the state of development of this field is still primitive, it would be premature to attempt the creation of a formal theory accounting for the relationship between dissociation and physical illness. I therefore review the relevant considerations and issues in a more informal manner, raising questions and considerations rather than proposing any unifying explanation.

DISSOCIATION AND PHYSICAL ILLNESS: CONCEPTUAL ISSUES

The DSM-IV (American Psychiatric Association 1994) definition of *dissociative disorders* is that the essential feature of these disorders is "a disruption in the usually integrated functions of consciousness, memory, identity, or perception of the environment" (American Psychiatric Association 1994, p. 477). This definition of dissociation causes a number of problems, which I will outline.

For historical reasons, the official definition of dissociation has been limited to those areas of the brain responsible for memory and identity (Ross 1989). This resulted in conversion disorder being classified as a somatoform disorder in DSM-III and DSM-III-R (American Psychiatric Association 1987) when it would have been more properly included among the dissociative disorders (Garcia 1990). Phenomenologically, conversion disorder is much more logically classified with psychogenic amnesia than with hypochondriasis. The DSM-III-R definition of dissociation was not consistent with the operationalized definition inherent in currently used measures of dissociation (see below), and its narrowness fostered the misclassification of conversion disorder as a somatoform disorder. The currently used inventories of dissociation inquire about dissociations of function from many areas of the brain; for instance, blocking out pain, hearing voices, and seeing someone else in the mirror are all dissociative phenomena inquired about in dissociative inventories and clinical assessments. The DSM-IV definition of conversion disorder requires the presence of "symptoms or deficits affecting voluntary motor or sensory function that suggest a neurological or general medical condition" (p. 452). It also requires an association of the symptoms with psychological factors and stressors in the absence of a detectable medical cause or evidence of malingering.

A phenomenologically based definition of dissociation, in contrast with the definition in DSM-IV, would be consistent with Braun's BASK (behavior, affect, sensation, knowledge) model of dissociation (Braun 1988a, 1988b). Braun's model is a summary of the clinical insight of the dissociative disorders field and assumes that dissociation can occur in any area of the brain. According to Braun's scheme, a pure dissociation of motor function is a conversion disorder, and a pure dissociation of memory is an instance of dissociative (psychogenic) amnesia. Both are properly classified as dissociative disorders. Unless such a clinical model or one similar to it is adopted as the foundation of discussion, it is difficult to see how dissociation could be relevant to physical illness and psychophysiology. There are complex relationships among hypnosis, dissociation, absorption, fantasy-proneness, somatization, and paranormal experiences, but no one phenomenon provides a complete explanation for any of the others; therefore, further research on these overlapping domains is likely to modify the definition of dissociation.

A second conceptual problem is the relationship between somatization disorder and dissociation. A recent review of somatization disorder does not mention childhood sexual abuse or dissociation despite review of a wide body of theory and research (Kellner 1990). In the one study, women with primary diagnoses of somatization disorder were asked about childhood sexual abuse; it was found that 60% provided such a history (Morrison 1989), of whom three were said on clinical grounds to have DID. I have conducted a number of studies in which somatization is linked to childhood trauma and other dissociative symptom clusters at high levels of significance in a variety of clinical populations and in the general population (C. A. Ross, unpublished observations, 1990; Ross et al. 1989a, 1989d; Ross et al. 1990a, 1990c).

Based on this body of research and review literature, I conclude that psychosomatic symptoms from all body systems are often dissociative in nature and related to chronic, severe childhood trauma. Research over the next decade may confirm that a large subgroup of patients with somatization disorder are best conceptualized as suffering from trauma disorders

(Ross 1989) and therefore are more properly grouped with the dissociative disorders than with somatoform disorders as conceptualized by Kellner in his 1990 review. If there is substance to the trauma model of somatization, a consensus on the relationship among dissociation, somatization, and trauma is required for planning of research projects, and research studying any of these variables in isolation from the others is not likely to be illuminating.

The next issue in this line of thinking is whether dissociation is linked to physiological changes occurring outside the central nervous system. The question, informally stated, is, "Are psychosomatic symptoms all in the head?" Even if psychosomatic symptoms are accepted as being dissociative and trauma related in many cases, that does not necessarily mean that they are accompanied by measurable changes in peripheral physiology.

One could hypothesize that extensive childhood sexual abuse can result in the medical symptom of dyspareunia, which is painful intercourse, and predict that in a woman with this psychosexual symptom there might be measurable abnormalities in pelvic floor muscle tone and vaginal lubrication on exposure to laboratory stimuli. These abnormalities in peripheral physiology might normalize with behavioral treatment or in some cases might require extensive uncovering psychotherapy. One could design studies with pre- and posttest measures of dissociation, physiological measures, and a well-documented psychotherapy that resulted in recovery of dissociated traumatic affect and memory, with resolution of symptoms. Until such studies are conducted, it will remain unknown whether dissociation and physical illness might be related through effects of trauma on peripheral physiology.

Future research might also involve attempts to demonstrate state-dependent physiological changes maintained by dissociative mechanisms. DID likely provides the best laboratory model for such studies (Putnam 1991), and positive findings in such studies would bring us closer to hard evidence of the psychophysiological reality of dissociation. Suggestive studies done to date have not yielded a substantial body of methodologically adequate and replicated data, and therefore no firm conclusions about the physiological reality of dissociation can be drawn at this time.

A final line of potential research is the most general one and consists of a series of interlinked questions: Is dissociation a common mechanism in nonpsychiatric physical illness, and if so does it promote health, illness, or both? Spiegel et al.'s (1989) finding that hypnosis appears to prolong survival of breast cancer patients offers highly suggestive evidence of a positive effect. Clinicians have been impressed at an anecdotal level by the ability of DID patients to regulate allergic responses, cardiac rhythms, and a host of physiological functions, but we do not know whether this ability can be systematically documented then harnessed for use in general medicine. Although very little is known about such possibilities, the intrinsic interest and potential clinical applications of any hard findings make this a worthwhile area of future investigation.

To summarize the issues and considerations to this point, further thinking, research, and discussion are required on the following:

1. Whether we should adopt a definition of dissociation encompassing all areas of the brain
2. Whether the dissociative response to trauma is a major pathway to somatization
3. Whether measurable dissociation-driven, state-dependent changes in psychophysiology can be demonstrated
4. Whether the dissociative modulation of peripheral physiology is likely to be of general medical relevance

---

MEASURES OF SOMATIZATION AND DISSOCIATION

The purpose of this section is to provide brief consideration of the self-report measures, structured interviews, and other inventories of potential use in research on dissociation and physical illness. There are only a few measures of dissociation to consider, because there are a relatively small number of investigators in this young field, and less work has been done than in other areas of psychiatry. The Dissociative Experiences Scale (DES; (Bernstein and Putnam 1986) is by far the most widely used, reliable, and valid self-report inventory. Another self-report measure of dissociation, the Perceptual Alteration Scale (Sanders 1986), has not been tested in clinical populations; therefore, it has no clinical reliability or validity. The Questionnaire of Experiences of Dissociation (Riley 1988) has promising psychometric properties, but no data are available other than the initial brief report describing its reliability and validity. The Dissociation Questionnaire developed in Belgium by Vanderlinden et al. (1991) appears to be a useful measure, and an English translation is available, but North American data are not yet available so its utility compared with the DES is unknown.

The DES can discriminate subjects with dissociative disorders from other diagnostic groups (Bernstein and Putnam 1986; Ross et al. 1988), general population norms and a factor structure are available (Ross et al. 1990b; Ross et al. 1991), and it has been used in a wide variety of studies reviewed by Dr. Carlson in Chapter 3 of this volume. The only limitation of the DES is that it has not yet been demonstrated to be sensitive to treatment outcome, although this will almost certainly prove to be the case. Studies of somatization and dissociation using the DES should take its factor structure into account because dissociation is clearly not a unitary phenomenon, and therefore relationships between physical illness and the three factors of the scale might be variable.

There are two structured interviews for diagnosing dissociative disorders: the Dissociative Disorders Interview Schedule (DDIS; Ross 1989; Ross et al. 1989c) and the Structured Clinical Interview for DSM-IV Dissociative Disorders (SCID-D; Steinberg et al. 1993). Both require further reliability and validation studies, but both have good initial reliability and validity for the diagnosis of DID. Dr. Steinberg describes the SCID-D in detail in Chapter 4 of this volume.

Both the DDIS and the SCID-D can be used for diagnostic purposes in research. Both contain internal subscales and/or symptom clusters that provide measures of the severity of dissociation and could potentially be used as state-change measures. As is true of the DES, this has not yet been demonstrated. Because Dr. Steinberg discusses the SCID-D in this volume, I will briefly describe the DDIS.

Advantages of the DDIS in somatization-dissociation research are that it includes all the DSM-III-R symptoms of somatization disorder plus a variety of dissociative symptom clusters; it gathers detailed information about childhood physical and sexual abuse; it documents prior psychiatric treatment; it can be administered in 30–45 minutes; it is easy to learn to administer; and general population norms for the DDIS are available as well as norms for different diagnostic groups, including schizophrenia, panic disorder, eating disorders, temporal lobe epilepsy, and substance abuse. The DDIS provides an economical way of gathering essential information in this line of research. A worthwhile strategy, given sufficient resources, would be to co-administer the DDIS and SCID-D in a series of studies that, along with the DES, would provide information on concurrent validity of the measures and a rich documentation of clinical dissociation.

Somatization is measured by a number of widely used instruments, but

I am not an expert on any of these and cannot offer an authoritative opinion. I have used a variety of measures in my own research, however, and will comment on them briefly.

The Symptom Checklist—90 (SCL-90) is a self-report measure of general psychopathology with nine subscales, one of which is called *somatization* (Derogatis et al. 1974). I have found this subscale to be sensitive to a history of trauma and to elevations on DES and DDIS dissociative symptom clusters. The advantages of the SCL-90 are that it is easy to administer and score, is very widely used, and also provides a general measure of psychopathology. Briere and Runtz (1990) have developed a dissociative subscale complementary to the SCL-90, which seems to be a good candidate for self-report measurement of dissociation and which might be added to any battery used in studies of dissociation and physical illness.

The Diagnostic Interview Schedule (DIS; Robins et al. 1981) contains a section for diagnosing somatization disorder, but the DIS is cumbersome to learn and administer and offers no advantages over the DDIS as a measure of somatization. However, its administration would provide documentation of a wide range of psychiatric diagnoses and would therefore widen the scope and implications of any future studies. Use of a structured interview like the DIS would likely be limited to studies with substantial funding because the interview training and hours involved are considerable.

The Minnesota Multiphasic Personality Inventory (MMPI; Hathaway and McKinley 1967) and the Millon Clinical Multiaxial Inventory (MCMI; Millon 1977) both provide information on somatization. I have used the MCMI and found that several of its subscales, including the somatoform subscale, are sensitive to dissociation and trauma. One of these two widely used inventories would provide a measure of personality disorder, extensive information about general psychopathology, and specific data on somatization and so therefore would be useful.

In summary, research on dissociation and physical illness should likely include a basic psychometric package consisting of the DES, DDIS and/or SCID-D, SCL-90, and MCMI or MMPI. This instrument battery would tap the major domains relevant to research on dissociation, somatization, and physical illness. Other measures of hypnotizability, absorption, and imaginative involvement might also be included depending on the special interests of investigators. Attention should be paid to the order of administration of the tests, the degree of blindness of the subjects to the rationale of the research, and the blindness of DDIS and SCID-D interviewers to other research and clinical data and to subject group membership.

RECENT RESEARCH ON DISSOCIATION
AND PHYSICAL ILLNESS

The trauma model of psychopathology predicts that traumatized subsets of most DSM-III-R diagnostic groups, including depression and schizophrenia, if appropriately studied, would exhibit distinct phenomenology, pathophysiology, family transmission, and response to psychotherapy and psychopharmacology (Ross 1991). Including a history of severe childhood sexual abuse as an exclusion criterion in trials of antidepressants might, if the model is correct, increase the medication response rate from 70% to 90% and reduce the placebo response rate from 35% to 20%. If this occurred, the specificity and efficacy of a new antidepressant medication could be demonstrated with substantially less development cost.

With respect to physical illness, the question is whether there is a large traumatic-dissociative subgroup within certain medical diagnoses. A second related question is whether traumatic pathways to dissociation are illustrated by certain medical illnesses. I will deal with the second question first.

Two disorders have been studied as possible biomedical models of dissociation with negative findings. Temporal lobe epilepsy (Loewenstein and Putnam 1988; Putnam 1986; Ross et al. 1989b) and multiple sclerosis (Ross et al. 1990c) do not produce dissociative symptoms to any significant degree, and both disorders can be differentiated from DID at high levels of significance using the DES and DDIS. The search for a biomedical model of clinical dissociation has been unfruitful to date, and I am not aware of any other candidate disorders that have been proposed for study; therefore, this line of investigation does not appear to be a high priority currently.

Two medical disorders/symptom complexes with large posttraumatic-dissociative subgroups that have been studied to date are irritable bowel syndrome (Drossman et al. 1990; Siemens and Ross 1991) and nonorganic pelvic pain (Walker et al. 1988). Rates of childhood sexual abuse are much higher in people with these problems than in the general population; therefore, individuals with these disorders should be good subjects for study of the relationship between dissociation and physical illness.

In our study (Siemens and Ross 1991), patients with irritable bowel syndrome had much higher rates of childhood sexual abuse and many more psychosomatic symptoms from a variety of body systems than patients in two other diagnostic groups: 1) patients with Crohn's disease or ulcerative colitis, and 2) patients with other gastrointestinal disorders, including peptic ulcer, hiatus hernia, bowel cancer, and gallbladder disease. These differences could not be accounted for by demographic variables and were highly specific because the three groups did not differ on a wide range of other symptom clusters using the DES, DDIS, and SCL-90.

The discovery of large groups of previously unrecognized trauma disorder patients in psychiatric clinical populations can apparently be generalized to at least some disorders in general medicine. It would be possible to design outcome studies of the psychotherapy of irritable bowel syndrome that took the sexual abuse into account, with medical symptoms serving as the treatment outcome measure, much like the studies of dyspareunia proposed earlier.

Other candidate medical illnesses should be identified for trauma-dissociation research, including perhaps gynecological and genitourinary disorders such as hyperemesis gravidarum, habitual abortion, ectopic pregnancy, dyspareunia, and urinary retention. The hypothesis concerning ectopic pregnancy is that childhood sexual abuse leads to promiscuity, which increases the risk for pelvic inflammatory disease, which in turn increases the risk for ectopic pregnancy, and the specific prediction is that women in their 20s with ectopic pregnancies should have higher rates of childhood sexual abuse and higher levels of dissociative symptomatology than control subjects.

Sexually transmitted diseases of all kinds are likely more common in individuals with trauma histories and elevated dissociation scores. In some disorders, a specific psychosomatic mechanism might be involved, whereas in others, such as AIDS, the disorder in a subgroup of individuals may be a consequence of trauma-driven behavior such as prostitution or intravenous drug abuse.

A number of other speculative possibilities are worthy of mention: Individuals who experience spontaneous remissions or long-term survival with serious malignancies might prove to be more hypnotizable or to have higher DES scores than those who fare less well. The spontaneous operation of healing dissociative mechanisms in such individuals might be subject to naturalistic documentation. Anecdotal clinical observation suggests, for instance, that some individuals with DID have very fast wound healing. If this is correct, it is a property of the human mind that might be subject to augmentation in non-DID individuals. It is possible that higher DES scores predict lower narcotic requirements in terminal malignancies because such individuals are better able to dissociate their pain on their own. This property of dissociation, if it exists, must be intertwined with hypnotizability.

In contrast, it might be possible to document deleterious effects of high dissociative capacity on the prevalence, course, and outcome of physical illness. An example of the disadvantage of being highly dissociative might be higher rates of delirium tremens or postoperative psychosis in high-scoring DES subjects than in relevant control subjects. In such cases, the *psychosis,* upon close examination, might prove to be more dissociative than psychotic in nature. The highly dissociative individual is perhaps more likely to manifest dissociative symptoms of delirium in response to the brain disturbance in alcohol withdrawal than is a person with low dissociative capacity.

There are many medical illnesses that might profitably be studied with the trauma-dissociation model. Subgroups within these disorders might respond to trauma-based psychotherapy or might provide insight into mechanisms that could be harnessed for general use throughout medicine. In some instances, such as AIDS or hepatitis acquired by sharing dirty needles, the relationship between trauma, dissociation, and the medical disorder might be indirect and mediated through behavior, but specific trauma-oriented psychotherapeutic interventions might still be beneficial. I mention the above speculations to illustrate the potential richness and clinical applications of research into dissociation and physical illness. As I stated at the beginning of this chapter, we are in the stage of documenting phenomenological linkages and proposing specific research studies, and it would be premature to attempt to construct a synthesizing theory at this time.

The linkages between trauma, dissociation, somatization, and pathophysiology, if they exist, probably take many forms and probably are mediated in many different ways. Unrecognized, long-term, dissociative consequences of childhood trauma may permeate society at all levels and may cost billions of dollars per year in lost productivity and medical and psychiatric care. Within general medicine, our failure to recognize and focus on the long-term consequences of severe childhood trauma may result in significant expenditures for tests and treatments that are ineffective and produce complications.

To summarize the ideas outlined in this section, relationships between dissociation and physical illness might take the following forms:

1. A direct relationship between psychological trauma and peripheral pathophysiology, as in dyspareunia
2. An effect of trauma mediated through behavior rather than through psychosomatic mechanisms, as in transmission of AIDS by dirty needles

3. Dissociation and childhood trauma increasing the risk for an illness both through behavior and through psychological/central nervous system mechanisms, as in delirium tremens (in some individuals, the alcoholism may be driven by childhood trauma and the withdrawal symptoms may be predominantly dissociative in nature)
4. High dissociative capacity correlated with spontaneous remission of malignancies
5. Trauma/dissociation altering the response to medications, for example, reducing narcotic requirements in terminal malignancy
6. State-dependent, dissociation-driven alterations in physiology: these might be harnessed for general use, for instance, in adjunctive control of cardiac arrhythmias
7. Amplification of immune surveillance mechanisms

These examples are included as an illustrative list of possible ways in which dissociation might interact with physical illness, although most are entirely speculative and are included primarily to stimulate thought. One research strategy would be to select candidate disorders with a high likelihood of positive findings and to study them using the measures discussed above. Although the trauma model focuses on psychopathology, it is essential to remember that dissociation is often normal and adaptive. It is possible that research of the kind discussed in this chapter could help bring psychiatry back into medicine more effectively than the currently dominant bioreductionist model of psychopathology. In conclusion, I want to emphasize once again that the purpose of this chapter is not to propose a formal theory but rather to communicate current thinking, research, speculation, and clinical observation within the dissociative disorders field concerning dissociation and physical illness.

REFERENCES

Alvarado CS: Dissociation and state-specific psychophysiology during the nineteenth century. Dissociation 3:160–168, 1989

American Psychiatric Association: Diagnostic and Statistical Manual of Mental Disorders, 3rd Edition. Washington DC, American Psychiatric Association, 1980

American Psychiatric Association: Diagnostic and Statistical Manual of Mental Disorders, 3rd Edition, Revised. Washington, DC, American Psychiatric Association, 1987

American Psychiatric Association: Diagnostic and Statistical Manual of Mental Disorders, 4th Edition. Washington, DC, American Psychiatric Association, 1994

Bernstein EM, Putnam FW: Development, reliability, and validity of a dissociation scale. J Nerv Ment Dis 174:727–735, 1986

Bliss EL: Multiple personalities: a report of 14 cases with implications for schizophrenia. Arch Gen Psychiatry 37:1399–1397, 1980

Braun BG: The BASK (behavior, affect, sensation, knowledge) model of dissociation. Dissociation 1:4–23, 1988a

Braun BG: The BASK model of dissociation: clinical applications. Dissociation 1:16–23, 1988b

Briere J, Runtz M: Augmenting Hopkins SCL scales to measure dissociative symptoms: data from two nonclinical samples. J Pers Assess 55:376–379, 1990

Coons PM: Multiple personality: diagnostic considerations. J Clin Psychiatry 41:330–336, 1980

Coons PM: Psychophysiologic investigations of multiple personality disorder. Dissociation 1:47–53, 1988

Derogatis LR, Lipman RS, Rickels K, et al: The Hopkins Symptom Checklist (HSCL): a self-report symptom inventory. Behav Sci 19:1–15, 1974

Drossman DS, Leserman J, Nachman G: Sexual and physical abuse in women with functional or organic gastrointestinal disorders. Ann Intern Med 113:828–833, 1990

Ellenberger HF: The Discovery of the Unconscious. New York, Basic Books, 1970

Garcia FO: The conception of dissociation and conversion in the new edition of the International Classification of Diseases (ICD-10). Dissociation 3:204–208, 1990

Goettman C, Greaves GB, Coons PM: Multiple Personality and Dissociation, 1791–1990: A Complete Bibliography. Atlanta, GA, George B Greaves, 1991

Greaves GM: Multiple personality disorder: 165 years after Mary Reynolds. J Nerv Ment Dis 168:577–596, 1980

Hathaway SR, McKinley JC: MMPI Manual. New York, Psychological Corporation, 1967

Hilgard ER: Divided Consciousness: Multiple Controls in Human Thought and Action. New York, Wiley, 1977

Kellner R: Somatization: theories and research. J Nerv Ment Dis 178:150–160, 1990

Loewenstein RJ: Somatoform disorders in victims of incest and child abuse, in Incest-Related Syndromes of Adult Psychopathology. Edited by Kluft RP. Washington, DC, American Psychiatric Press, 1990, pp 75–107

Loewenstein RJ, Putnam FW: A comparison study of dissociative symptoms in patients with complex partial seizures, multiple personality disorder, and posttraumatic stress disorder. Dissociation 1:17–23, 1988

Ludwig AM, Bradsma JM, Wilbur CB, et al: The objective study of a case of multiple personality, or, are four heads better than one? Arch Gen Psychiatry 26:298–310, 1972

Millon T: Millon Clinical Multiaxial Inventory Manual. Minneapolis, MN, National Cumputer Systems, 1977

Morrison J: Childhood sexual histories of women with somatization disorder. Am J Psychiatry 146:239–241, 1989

Putnam FW: The psychophysiologic investigation of multiple personality disorder: a review. Psychiatr Clin North Am 7:31–41, 1984

Putnam FW: The scientific investigation of multiple personality disorder, in Split Minds, Split Brains. Edited by Quen JM. New York, New York University Press, 1986, pp 109–125

Putnam FW: Diagnosis and Treatment of Multiple Personality Disorder. New York, Guilford, 1989

Putnam FW: Recent research on multiple personality disorder. Psychiatr Clin North Am 14:489–502, 1991

Riley KC: Measurement of dissociation. J Nerv Ment Dis 176:449–450, 1988

Robins LN, Helzer JE, Croughan J, et al: National Institute of Mental Health Diagnostic Interview Schedule. Arch Gen Psychiatry 38:381–389, 1981

Rosenbaum M: The role of the term schizophrenia in the decline of diagnoses of multiple personality. Arch Gen Psychiatry 37:1383–1385, 1980

Ross CA: Multiple Personality Disorder: Diagnosis, Clinical Features, and Treatment. New York, Wiley, 1989

Ross CA: Epidemiology of multiple personality disorder and dissociation. Psychiatr Clin North Am 14:503–517, 1991

Ross CA, Norton GR, Anderson G: The dissociative experiences scale: a replication study. Dissociation 1:21–22, 1988

Ross CA, Heber S, Norton GR, et al: Differences between multiple personality disorder and other diagnostic groups on structured interview. J Nerv Ment Dis 179:487–491, 1989a

Ross CA, Heber S, Anderson G, et al: Differentiating multiple personality disorder and complex partial seizures. Gen Hosp Psychiatry 11:54–58, 1989b

Ross CA, Heber S, Norton GR, et al: The dissociative disorders interview schedule: a structured interview. Dissociation 2:169–189, 1989c

Ross CA, Heber S, Norton GR, et al: Somatic symptoms in multiple personality disorder. Psychosomatics 30:154–160, 1989d

Ross CA, Anderson G, Heber S, et al: Dissociation and abuse in multiple personality patients, prostitutes, and exotic dancers. Hosp Community Psychiatry 41:328–330, 1990a

Ross CA, Joshi S, Currie RP: Dissociative experiences in the general population. Am J Psychiatry 147:1547–1552, 1990b

Ross CA, Fast E, Anderson G, et al: Somatic symptoms in multiple sclerosis and MPD. Dissociation 3:102–106, 1990c

Ross CA, Joshi S, Currie RP: Dissociation in the general population: identification of three factors. Hosp Community Psychiatry 42:297–301, 1991

Sanders S: The perceptual alteration scale: a scale measuring dissociation. Am J Clin Hypn 29:95–102, 1986

Siemens JG, Ross CA: Childhood sexual abuse and somatic symptoms in patients with gastrointestinal disorders, in Proceedings of the Eighth International Conference on Multiple Personality/Dissociative States. Edited by Braun BG, Carlson EB. Chicago, IL, Rush-Presbyterian-St. Luke's Medical Center, 1991, p 86

Spiegel D, Bloom JR, Kraemer HC, et al: Effect of psychosocial treatment on survival of patients with metastatic breast cancer. Lancet 2:888–891, 1989

Steinberg M: Structured Clinical Interview for DSM-IV dissociative disorders (SCID-D). Washington, DC, American Psychiatric Press, 1993

van der Kolk BA, van der Hart O: Pierre Janet and the breakdown of psyhological adaptation in psychological trauma. Am J Psychiatry 146:1530–1540, 1989

Vanderlinden J, Van Dyck R, Vandereycken MD, et al: Dissociative experiences in the general population in the Netherlands and Belgium: a study with the Dissociative Questionnaire (DIS-Q). Dissociation 4:180–184, 1991

Walker E, Katon W, Harrop-Griffiths J, et al: Relationship of chronic pelvic pain to psychiatric diagnoses and childhood sexual abuse. Am J Psychiatry 145:75–80, 1988

CHAPTER 8

Physiological Correlates of Hypnosis and Dissociation

David Spiegel, M.D., and Eric Vermutten M.D.

ypnotic and dissociative states have long been associated with unusual effects on the body, ranging from raising blisters to eliminating warts, although a neurophysiological signature of these states themselves has remained elusive. They may be best conceptualized as necessary but not sufficient conditions within which individuals may optimize their control over certain perceptual, motor, and autonomic processes.

Dissociation is a separation of mental events that would ordinarily be processed together—a discontinuity of memory, identity, perception, motor function, or consciousness. Dissociation may, for example, involve differences in perception of similar sensations from one part of the body compared with another. Alternatively, there may be a sense of involuntariness associated with movement, as though parts of the body were governed by different motor control systems. For example, in hypnosis instructed movement is usually performed with a sense of involuntariness (Spiegel and Spiegel 1978/1987; Weitzenhoffer 1980). This dissociated movement feels as if it were happening on its own, independent of customary volition and control. Such dissociative phenomena may be formally induced with hypnosis but also occur spontaneously.

Clinically, more extreme forms of dissociation than those elicited under formal hypnosis occur. An example is dissociative amnesia, in which one period of time is dissociated in memory from the general continuity in memory of personal history. A Vietnam combat veteran, for example, developed an inability to recall the narrative facts of a period of time following the death of a child he had informally adopted, despite having been conscious at the time and remembering it immediately afterward (Spiegel 1981). Another example is dissociative identity disorder (DID; formerly called multiple personality disorder), in which different personality states, each with its own partially independent sets of memories, coexist in the same person and vie for control of consciousness. (Dr. Ross reviews evidence of physiological differences observed across personalities in DID in Chapter 7.)

This dissociative compartmentalization of experience is accomplished through a complementary focusing of attention. Hypnotic and dissociative phenomena may be understood to be a clarifying extreme of human attentional processes (Hilgard 1977; Spiegel 1988). *Hypnosis* is at one end of the continuum of attention, involving an enhancement in focal concentration with a relative suspension of peripheral awareness (Spiegel and Spiegel 1978/1987). Hypnotic concentration is analogous to looking through a telephoto lens in a camera. What one sees is detailed, but the field of vision is narrow. *Absorption* is a tendency to become fully involved in a perceptual imaginative or ideational experience (Tellegen 1981; Tellegen and Atkinson 1974). There is evidence that individuals prone to this type of cognition are more high-hypnotizable than those who never fully engage in such experiences. *Hypnotic absorption* is a mental state in which cognitive resources are fully allocated to the central task, with little in the way of distraction. Information that is not at the focus of attention is kept well out of consciousness (i.e., dissociated from conscious awareness). The more highly focused attention is on a central percept or thought, the more likely that all other material is kept out of conscious awareness (i.e., dissociated; Spiegel 1990).

Hypnosis can be understood as controlled and structured dissociation, a normal microdissociative episode (Nemiah 1985; Spiegel and Spiegel 1978/1987). Thus hypnosis provides a model system for exploring the neurophysiological and somatic correlates of dissociative processes. There are several advantages of the hypnotic state: the relative unity of attentional focus and reliable trait differences (Piccione and Hilgard 1989; Spiegel and Spiegel 1978/1987). These enable experimental comparisons between *low*- and *high-hypnotizable* individuals attempting to perform the same tasks as well as comparisons between high-hypnotizable individuals in and out of formal hypnosis. In this chapter, electrophysiological studies relevant to the brain basis of hypnosis and dissociative processes are examined, followed by a review of the literature on effects of hypnosis and dissociation on somatic functions.

NEUROPHYSIOLOGY OF HYPNOSIS

Power Spectral Analysis

Power spectral analysis of the electroencephalogram (EEG) is an examination of the relative power of different frequency bands recorded across the scalp with the subject in a resting condition. It has potential utility in the characterization and localization of brain activity associated with hypnotic states. Initially, there was evidence of a greater tendency of high-hypnotizable subjects to generate alpha patterns, especially over the left compared with the right cerebral hemisphere (Morgan et al. 1974). The hypnotizability of the subjects was more strongly associated with these alpha patterns than whether the subjects were formally induced into a state of hypnosis. It was thus a trait rather than a state finding.

The meaning of a predominance of alpha power over a given brain region is unclear. It is commonly interpreted as the noise the brain makes when it is alert but doing little, analogous to an engine idling. For example, alpha power is typically increased over the occipital cortex when an alert subject closes his or her eyes. Thus the relative preponderance of alpha over the left compared with the right cerebral hemisphere was interpreted by the Hilgard group as indicating greater activity in the right cerebral hemisphere. However, subsequent research has not supported this finding (Lubar et al. 1991; Sabourin et al. 1990). Edmonston and Moscovitz (1990), using overall EEG power as the criterion, reported that the right hemisphere is not selectively activated in hypnosis. Recent research has shown higher levels of theta activity among high-hypnotizable subjects, especially in frontal leads, during hypnosis (Sabourin et al. 1990). Also, De Pascalis et al. (1989) found higher EEG density in the 40 Hz range among high-hypnotizable and hypnotized subjects during an emotional recall task. During recall of negative emotions, this EEG density was higher over the right compared with the left cerebral hemisphere. During recall of positive emotions, 40 Hz density was higher on both sides. This finding is congruent with research showing an association between positive emotionality and the functioning of the left frontal pole, and negative emotionality and the functioning of the right frontal pole (Davidson et al. 1990; Kinsbourne 1988). For example, damage to the left frontal region caused by a cerebrovascular accident tends to produce a catastrophic reaction, perhaps due to the unopposed activity of the right frontal pole. Conversely, damage to the right frontal cortex is

associated with indifference. Thus, the literature on power spectral correlates of hypnosis is limited, with interest shifting away from alpha to other
frequency bands.

Event-Related Potentials

Cortical event-related potentials (ERPs) have been widely employed in
studying perceptual processing (Donchin et al. 1978; Pritchard 1981). ERPs
are averaged EEGs time locked to the presentation of a series of stimuli.
This method provides excellent temporal resolution by assessing scalp-
recorded response to stimuli within a time frame of approximately 500
milliseconds. Thus this method has the advantage of providing good control
over cognitive processes occurring in response to stimuli, unlike newer
brain imaging techniques, such as positron-emission tomography (PET),
which have temporal resolution ranging from 40 seconds to 30 minutes.
However, the spatial localization of ERPs is not as good because electrical
activity is propagated throughout brain tissue and the scalp, making localization of the precise sources of waveforms difficult, although new localization algorithms have been developed recently.

Early and late components of the waveform are to some extent differ-
entially influenced by external (exogenous) and internal (endogenous) factors. The amplitude of early components (100–200 milliseconds after stimuli
are presented) primarily reflects input signal intensity and the type of signal
(e.g., visual versus auditory; Ford et al. 1978; Hillyard and Picton 1979;
Sutton et al. 1965). The amplitude of later components (200–500 milliseconds after the stimulus is presented) is increased by novelty (Baribeau-
Braun et al. 1983; Duncan-Johnson and Donchin 1980; Hillyard and Picton
1978; Johnson 1980; Pritchard 1981; Sutton et al. 1965), conscious awareness of the signals (Posner 1978; Posner et al. 1973), and task relevance
(Pritchard 1981; Squires et al. 1975). Thus early amplitude is most influenced by the nature of that which is perceived; later components are most
influenced by the perceiver.

This body of ERP research provides a natural framework for testing the
neurophysiology of hypnosis and dissociation. Hypnotically induced alterations in perceptual processing, such as the reduction or elimination of pain
to the production of visual and auditory hallucinations, should be accompanied by changes in the amplitude of ERPs beyond that seen through
conventional attention manipulations. For example, when instructed to
block or reduce perception of a stimulus in hypnosis, one should see a

reduction in ERP amplitude to those stimuli and conversely. Half of the early studies did demonstrate such a relationship between a hypnotic reduction in perception and ERP amplitude reduction (Clynes et al. 1964; Galbraith et al. 1972; Guerrero-Figueroa and Heath 1964; Hernandez-Peon and Donoso 1959; N. J. Wilson 1968). One early study of hypnotizability in relationship to ERPs demonstrated that high-hypnotizable individuals were more successful at focusing attention and filtering out unwanted stimuli, for example, reduced ERP amplitude in an unattended sensory modality (Galbraith et al. 1972). Interestingly, low-hypnotizable individuals showed the opposite effect, an increased amplitude of response to signals that were supposed to be filtered out, suggesting a limitation in the ability to deploy focal rather than peripheral attention.

However, numerous other early studies failed to demonstrate any relationship between hypnotic perceptual alteration and ERP changes (Amadeo and Yanovski 1975; Andreassi et al. 1976; Beck and Barolin 1965; Beck et al. 1966; Halliday and Mason 1964; Serafetinides 1968; Zakrzewski and Szelenberger 1981). This body of research was limited by small samples, the use of psychiatrically and neurologically ill patients rather than normal populations, qualitative rather than quantitative analysis of ERP amplitude, and confusing hypnotic instructions. For example, telling a hypnotized person to reduce the intensity of a stimulus rather than ignore it is paradoxical. It requires attending to the stimulus for the purpose of reducing its intensity, which could enhance rather than diminish cortical response to it (Spiegel and Barabasz 1988, 1990).

Recent studies have demonstrated ERP amplitude changes consistent with the content of hypnotic hallucinations in visual, somatosensory, and auditory systems (Sigalowitz et al. 1991; Spiegel et al. 1985; Spiegel et al. 1989). Effects of hypnosis have been observed primarily in the endogenous or late components of the ERP, the P_{300}. For example, there was significant P_{300} reduction across the scalp to visual stimuli when high-hypnotizable subjects were instructed that there was a hallucinated cardboard box blocking their view of the stimulus-generating monitor. Low-hypnotizable subjects given the same instructions showed no such difference (see Figure 8–1). This effect was stronger over the right than with the left occipital cortex (Spiegel et al. 1985).

Similar alteration in ERP amplitude congruent with hypnotic perceptual alteration has also been found when somatosensory stimuli are used (Spiegel et al. 1989; see Figure 8–2). The hypnotic instruction is analogous to that used clinically for pain control. Subjects were told that their hand would be cool and numb and that this numbness would filter out any other sensations in the affected area. There was a significant reduction in the P_{300} amplitude and also in the P_{100} amplitude, suggesting earlier filtering of this somatosensory signal in the hypnotic hallucination condition. Thus these

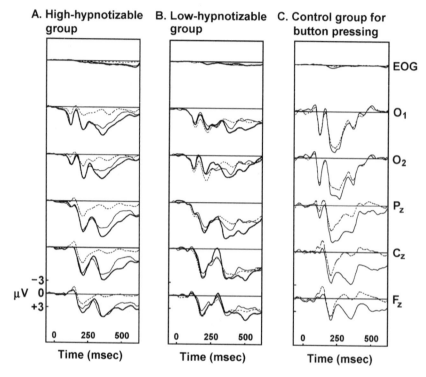

Figure 8–1. Effect of hypnotic obstructive hallucination on visual evoked potentials. Visual evoked potentials (VEPs) recorded at leads F_z, C_z, P_z, O_1, and O_2 are expressed as the mean of recordings in each condition from six individuals per group yielding approximately 1,800 VEPs per waveform. In *A* and *B*, high-hypnotizable and low-hypnotizable group data shown are VEPs to stimuli observed in the hypnotic enhancement condition *(thick solid lines),* the hypnotic diminution condition *(thin solid lines),* and the hypnotic obstructive hallucination condition *(dotted lines).* In *C,* control subjects for button pressing, *solid lines* are VEPs to stimuli that were all treated as button-pressing targets. *Dotted lines* are VEPs in a passive attention condition in which all stimuli were treated as standards and required no button pressing.
Source. From Spiegel D, Cutcomb S, Ren C, et al.: "Hypnotic Hallucination Alters Evoked Potentials." *Journal of Abnormal Psychology* 94:249–255, 1985.
Copyright 1985 by the American Psychological Association. Reprinted by permission of the publisher.

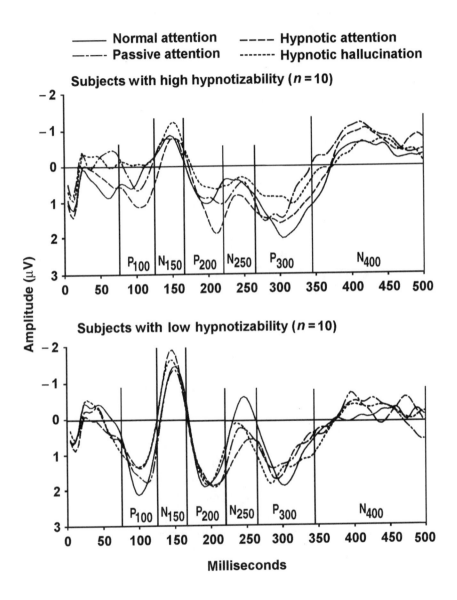

Figure 8–2. Mean amplitudes of somatosensory event-related potentials in four conditions for subjects with high and low hypnotizability.
Source. Reprinted with permission from Spiegel D, Bierre P, Rootenberg J: "Hypnotic Alteration of Somatosensory Perception." *American Journal of Psychiatry* 146:749–754, 1989.

subjects responded cortically as though the stimulus was less intense as well as less relevant. In another condition, subjects were told that the stimuli were pleasant and interesting and that they should pay full attention to them. This yielded a significant increase in P_{100} but not P_{300} amplitude in hypnosis. Thus high-hypnotizable subjects were capable of producing bidirectional changes in ERP amplitude to sensory stimuli, depending on the cognitive task employed during hypnosis. Low-hypnotizable subjects showed no such changes, although they were put through the identical set of instructions by an experimenter blind to their hypnotizability.

Recently, Zachariae and Bjerring (1990) administered a histamine subcutaneous injection to 10 high-hypnotizable subjects and gave hypnotic analgesia instructions while recording ERPs and found significant reductions in them during the analgesia condition. In addition, they found a significant difference in the histamine flare area, with a smaller flare reported in the hypnotic analgesia condition. This group has also observed an effect of hypnotically induced emotion on somatosensory ERPs (Zachariae et al. 1991).

Similar results have recently been obtained in the auditory system. Sigalowitz et al. (1991) found P_{300} differences among high-hypnotizable subjects hallucinating a reduction or increase in tones, whereas low-hypnotizable subjects did not show such a change. The amplitude reduction did not reach statistical significance but the increase during positive hallucination did.

Brain Imaging

There has been little study of hypnosis using newer brain imaging techniques such as PET, single photon emission computed tomography (SPECT), and magnetic resonance imaging (MRI). One study using PET demonstrated a global 16% increase in cerebral perfusion during hypnosis but no change during autogenic training in 12 normal subjects (Ulich et al. 1987).

These techniques have proven useful in identifying subsystems within the brain devoted to specific types of perceptual and cognitive processing, for example, activation of the left inferior frontal cortex and anterior cingulate gyrus in response to visual and auditory presentation of words (Volkow and Tancredi 1991). This brain imaging work has led to the parsing of attentional processes into a series of components with different neuroanatomical localizations, using PET imaging of brain responses to various attentional tasks (Posner and Peterson 1990). The posterior attentional system involves orienting with activation of the posterior prestriate cortex. Focusing of attention, such as the ability to detect a faint blip on a radar screen, is associated with activity in the anterior cingulate gyrus. Arousal involves activity in the right frontal cortex. These interesting new theories and the data that support them offer the possibility of greater specificity in identifying the neurophysiological basis of hypnotic processes. For example, the majority of observations of a connection between hypnosis and alteration in ERP amplitude have involved changes in the P_{300}, which are maximal over the frontal and central cortex. This would suggest some specific involvement of the anterior attentional systems in hypnotic concentration. These systems involve focusing (anterior cingulate) and arousal (frontal, especially on the right) phenomena that are consistent with the fact that hypnosis involves intense absorption, or focal attention, and is state of resting alertness or arousal. On the other hand, hypnotic perceptual alteration involves the primary association cortices as well.

Neurotransmitters

Further indirect evidence for the involvement of the frontal cortex in hypnotic phenomena derives from a recent finding that hypnotizability is significantly correlated with cerebrospinal fluid levels of homovanillic acid (HVA), a metabolite of dopamine (Spiegel and King 1992). Levels of HVA in the cerebrospinal fluid primarily reflect activity in the frontal cortex and basal ganglia, regions rich in dopaminergic synapses. Administration of amphetamine, which stimulates the release of dopamine, has been shown to enhance hypnotizability (Sjoberg and Hollister 1965). Although at first the basal ganglia might seem irrelevant to such attention deployment mechanisms, the automaticity observed in hypnotic motor behavior could represent an activation of this region, which is involved in both implicit memory (Mishkin 1991; Schacter 1987) and routine motor activity, especially of large muscle groups.

Summary

A great deal remains to be learned about the possible neuroanatomical and neurophysiological correlates of hypnotic and dissociative states. Although efforts to determine a neurophysiological signature of the hypnotic state have been, in general, unrewarding, there does seem to be accumulating evidence that hypnotized individuals have an unusual ability to modify neurophysiological processing of perceptions. Electrophysiological and neurochemical evidence suggests special roles of the frontal and temporal lobes, with mixed evidence regarding the predominance of the right cerebral hemisphere in hypnotic and dissociative states. Recent brain imaging work on attention suggests that hypnotic concentration may involve activation of centers in the anterior cingulate gyrus and the right frontal lobe. Recent data on the relationship between levels of a dopamine metabolite and hypnotizability suggest a possible role for the frontal lobes and the basal ganglia in hypnotic phenomena. There is reason to hope that further research in this area, especially coupled with newer functional brain imaging techniques, may provide more evidence regarding the neurophysiological basis of hypnotic and dissociative states. This research also shows that high-hypnotizable individuals have an unusually good capacity to alter perception, both subjectively and objectively. This should be reflected in changes of peripheral somatic functions as well as central neurophysiological processing.

DISSOCIATION, HYPNOSIS, AND SOMATIC FUNCTION

Hypnotic and dissociative states have long been observed to be associated with heightened mental control over physical processes. This makes sense, given that attention is focused and distraction is minimized. Whatever the resources for cognitive control over the body, they should be maximally mobilized during hypnotic concentration. The classic example is pain control. It has been known since the middle of the last century that hypnosis is quite effective in reducing, or at times eliminating, even severe pain (Esdaile 1957; Hilgard and Hilgard 1975; Spiegel 1985/1986). In addition, hypnosis has been shown to be effective in eliminating warts (Sinclair-Geiben and Chalmers 1959; Spanos et al. 1988; Surman et al. 1973), controlling gastric acid secretion (Klein and Spiegel 1989), and controlling symptoms of irritable bowel syndrome (Whorwell et al. 1984).

There is a substantial literature, albeit often anecdotal, documenting various effects of hypnosis on physical function. The literature seems to support several statements about hypnosis: 1) that high-hypnotizable individuals seem to have a special ability to translate mental events into physical effects, one which is not always within their conscious control, and 2) effects of hypnosis on bodily functions seem more prominent among visible bodily parts available to consciousness, especially the skin.

It must be borne in mind that there is a general tendency to publish positive findings and submit negative ones to the circular file. The best available reports of effects of hypnosis on various somatic functions must be viewed not necessarily as the tip of the iceberg but rather as a nonrandom sampling of phenomena. At the same time, one well-done controlled study, or several astute clinical observations, can serve to document that an interesting and robust phenomenon exists. The interested reader is referred to a thoughtful review by Theodore X. Barber (1961) and to a review of medical effects of hypnosis by Frankel (1987).

RISKS AND BENEFITS OF HIGH HYPNOTIZABILITY

High-hypnotizable individuals seem to be vulnerable to conversion disorders, suggesting that hypnotic states may be mobilized spontaneously to produce pseudosomatic conversion symptoms. In their review of the special characteristics of high-hypnotizable individuals, S. C. Wilson and Barber (1981, 1983) made the startling observation that 60% of their sample had experienced pseudocyesis, with symptoms that included amenorrhea, breast changes, and abdominal enlargement. One of their subjects had had a hysterical illness that had been misdiagnosed as rheumatic fever, complete with an elevated sedimentation rate. These subjects also experienced dramatic physical symptoms stimulated by stress. For example, many of them reported being physically nauseated by violence in the movies.

Similarly, Apfel et al. (1986) reported that patients with hyperemesis gravidarum who had severe symptoms ($n = 17$) were significantly more hypnotizable on the Stanford Hypnotic Clinical scale than those who had only moderate symptoms ($n = 13$). Pettinati and Wade (1986) studied 86 patients with eating disorders. The 21 patients with bulimia had a mean Stanford Hypnotic Susceptibility Scale–Form C score of 7.71, significantly higher than anorexic patients with purging symptoms ($n = 46$), who scored 6.1, and anorexic patients who were solely abstainers ($n = 19$), whose hypnotizability scores were only 5.0. This finding is similar to the observation of Andreychuk and Skriver (1975) of a correlation between the severity of migraine headache symptoms and hypnotizability. They had originally set out to demonstrate that hypnotizability predicted better response to a variety of treatments, which they also found. But this and other studies indicate that hypnotizability is a two-edged sword and that high-hypnotizable individuals are likely to use their intensified mind-body relatedness unwittingly as a means of experiencing and expressing conflict.

HYPNOTIC EFFECTS ON SKIN DISORDERS

There are some 10 studies documenting positive effects of hypnosis in eliminating warts. The classic study was done by Sinclair-Gieben and Chalmers (1959). Fourteen subjects were hypnotized and told that the warts would be eliminated on only one-half of their body. Nine of these subjects responded with elimination of warts on only the designated part of the body. Another 5 did not respond. Surman et al. (1973) attempted to replicate this finding, adding to the methodology a control group who had no intervention. Nine of the 17 responded, but 8 of the 9 responded on both sides of the body, thus failing to replicate the somatic specificity observed in the earlier study. Of more interest, however, is that none of the control patients reported elimination of their warts. Recently, Spanos et al. (1990) reported that subjects who were hypnotized lost significantly more warts than no-treatment controls at 6-week follow-up, whereas those administered topical salicylic acid and those offered a placebo showed no such improvement. This study is of interest because Spanos and his group published a large number of studies attempting to debunk the specific effect of hypnosis and emphasizing the effects of social influence and patient expectation (Spanos 1986; Spanos and Hewett 1980; Spiegel 1985/1986, 1987), including their own earlier work on warts (Spanos et al. 1988).

Hypnosis has been shown to be effective in treating other chronic and more severe skin diseases—for example, psoriasis. Frankel and Misch (1973) reported a dramatic cure of a patient with a 20-year history of long-standing severe psoriasis after teaching the patient to use self-hypnosis to imagine himself in a warm, dry environment. However, Frankel (1987) later observed that therapeutic efforts in three subsequent cases were not successful. Surman and Crumpacker (1987) reported that hypnotic suggestion for genital herpes simplex resulted in only moderate treatment responses. There are five clinical reports of success in the use of hypnosis in treating

have reported modification of the delayed hypersensitivity response with hypnosis. In one well-done study, Ikemi and Nakagawa (1962) used hypnosis with five students and nonhypnotic suggestion with another eight students, and in one condition suggested that they were being touched with a poison ivy–type leaf when in fact they were being touched with a harmless leaf. All subjects in both conditions developed some degree of inflammation to the harmless leaf. In the second part of the study, the deception was reversed. They were told they were being touched with a harmless leaf and in fact were touched with the antigenic leaf. Only one subject in each group developed an inflammatory reaction in this condition. Several other studies (Black 1963a; Mason 1960) show that hypnosis could inhibit a previously demonstrated response to tuberculin. Black (1963b) showed decreased allergenic response in 8 of 12 subjects compared with the normal response. Fry et al. (1964) provided an interesting gradation of response in that they were able to show that three of nine subjects selected for some, but not high, hypnotizability could produce a suggested decrease in response to an allergenic stimulus at low, but not high, concentrations. There has been general agreement in this literature that higher hypnotizability favors greater ability to suppress delayed hypersensitivity responses (Mason 1963), although there is a more recent report that hypnotic suggestion did not alter delayed hypersensitivity (Locke et al. 1987). However, Zachariae et al. (1989) demonstrated a mean reduction of 41% in erythema after a histamine test following hypnotic suggestion among eight highly hypnotizable individuals. They also found a significant difference (increase or decrease) in induration in response to purified protein derivative in the left compared with the right arm following hypnotic suggestion. Thus several, though not all, studies indicate a hypnotic effect on cellular immunity. In another experiment, Zachariae and Bjerring (1993) administered an antigenic challenge, dinitrochlorobenzene (DNCB) and diphenylcyclopropenone (DCP), to 16 subjects who were given hypnotic suggestions to increase and decrease their response. One group was told to increase reactions to DNCB and decrease reactions to DCP, and another group was given the opposite instruction. Visual scoring blind to condition demonstrated a significant difference, and there was a clearly significant difference in skin thickness. This experiment suggests that hypnotic instruction may influence the magnitude of the hypersensitivity reaction.

One study provides evidence for a hypnotic effect on humoral immunity as well. Olness et al. (1989) gave specific hypnotic suggestions to children involving imagery that would increase immune substances in their saliva and compared salivary immunoglobulin A (IgA) and immunoglobulin G (IgG) levels after this and other hypnotic suggestions. There was a significant increase in IgA but not IgG after the specific enhancing but not other hypnotic instructions. This study is intriguing, but salivary immunoglobulin levels are quite sensitive to dilution factors; therefore, they could appear to be increased by a decrease in the volume of salivary secretion, although the fact that only IgA and not IgG was increased mitigates this concern.

Psychoneuroimmunology is a complex and growing field. A variety of social factors, such as social isolation and stress (Glaser and Kiecolt-Glaser 1987; Glaser et al. 1985, 1986), have been shown to influence aspects of cellular immunity. It is also clear that the nervous system influences the immune system via neurotransmitters that find receptors on lymphocytes and that the immune system in turn influences the central nervous system via cytokines. This is an intriguing area for future research. Hypnotic effects on immune function are not unique but may be more focused and specific.

BLOOD FLOW

What is the mechanism by which such effects might be mediated? Clearly, it is likely an interaction of the nervous system, especially the autonomic nervous system, which innervates smooth muscle in arterioles, and the circulatory system, because, as noted above, there often seem to be differences in skin temperature, a phenomenon that has been documented with hypnosis (Grabowska 1971; Zimbardo et al. 1970). In these studies, hypnotized individuals have been shown to be able to alter skin temperature in one hand but not the other as much as 7°C. In one study, changes in core temperature were controlled and skin temperature rose, whereas rectal temperature declined in four of seven high-hypnotizable subjects (Raynaud et al. 1984). This observation of hypnotic control of skin temperature has been applied clinically in observations that hypnotized subjects are able to reduce or eliminate bleeding—for example, patients with hemophilia (Dubin and Shapiro 1974; Hanford et al. 1980; Swirsky-Sacchetti and Margolis 1986). The latter was a larger scale study with 30 subjects. Although LeBaw (1975) reported lower blood product use among eight patients with hemophilia who were taught self-hypnosis compared with 10 control subjects, sample bias may account for at least some of the difference (LeBaron and

Zeltzer 1984). There have been reports of success with other diseases such as an upper gastrointestinal hemorrhage (Bishay et al. 1984) and von Willebrand's disease (Fung and Lazar 1983) as well. This literature has been reviewed by LeBaron and Zeltzer (1984).

GASTROINTESTINAL SYSTEM

There have been fewer reports of hypnotic effects on other organ systems. However, there are several studies of the gastrointestinal system that indicate that hypnosis can facilitate an enhancement of cognitive control over physiological function. Whorwell et al. (1984) reported a well-conducted randomized trial showing that 15 patients with irritable bowel syndrome, treated with hypnosis, reported significant improvement in pain, abdominal distention, and diarrhea, as well as emotional well-being, compared with a control group of 15 patients. An 18-month follow-up of 15 of these patients showed continued remission, and they reported similar improvement in 35 additional patients. They noted that all patients under the age of 50 responded, contrasted with only one quarter of those over 50. Similarly, Zeltzer et al. (1984) reported significant reduction in symptoms among 19 patients taught hypnosis to control nausea and vomiting secondary to chemotherapy. However, the results in this study were uncorrelated with hypnotizability.

Klein and Spiegel (1989) observed significant hypnotic control of gastric acid secretion among 28 high-hypnotizable subjects. When hypnotized and instructed to eat an imaginary meal, basal acid output rose 89%. In a second study, subjects were instructed to use hypnosis to experience deep relaxation not involving hunger or eating and drinking. There was a significant 39% reduction in basal acid output. In a third trial, subjects were given an injection of pentagastrin, which stimulates maximal parietal cell output. There was a significant 11% reduction in pentagastrin-stimulated peak acid output. This study further emphasizes the two-edged sword aspect of high hypnotizability in that it facilitated bidirectional changes depending on mental content during the hypnotic state. That these observations may have clinical relevance is illustrated by a controlled trial of hypnosis in relapse prevention of duodenal ulcers (Colgan et al. 1988). Thirty patients with rapidly relapsing ulcer disease were randomly assigned, after ranitidine, to hypnosis or no treatment. All of the control patients but only 53% of the hypnosis patients relapsed. Thus hypnosis seems to be an effective adjunct to the management of some gastrointestinal disorders.

NEUROLOGICAL AND RESPIRATORY SYMPTOMS

There have been several anecdotal reports of hypnotic control of neurological symptoms, such as reduction in parkinsonian tremor (Wain et al. 1990) and the symptoms of Guillain-Barré syndrome, including an increase in muscle function (Sampson 1990). There have also been numerous reports of the effectiveness of hypnosis in controlling the symptoms of asthma (Collison 1968, 1975; Maher-Loughnan et al. 1962). These studies show a relationship between informally measured hypnotic capacity and responsiveness to treatment.

A high-hypnotizable patient with pigmentary glaucoma (Spiegel and Spiegel 1978/1987) found that her ocular pressure was directly proportional to stress in her life and that she could quickly learn to reduce it with training and self-hypnosis. She also observed that she was vulnerable to other somatic expressions of distress. For example, she found that when her mother-in-law was being exceedingly critical, she experienced a sudden loss of auditory acuity. She reflected later, "I just didn't want to hear what she was telling me." This patient may typify the kind of person who has *somatic absorption* (Barsky and Wyshak 1990) and thereby frequently translates emotional distress into somatic terms. It is also clear that high-hypnotizable individuals have considerable vividness of mental imagery and considerable control over their imagery (Perry 1973; Sheehan 1979; Shor et al. 1966; Spanos et al. 1973).

It has been reported that patients with dissociative disorders show fluctuations in physical symptoms when in different dissociative states. For example, a 29-year-old woman with DID and legal blindness from a birth injury had resting nystagmus and on visual testing her acuity was worse than 20/200. She could identify shapes but had little distance vision and used a Seeing Eye dog. She noted, however, that when a child alter personality had been in control, she had been able to recognize people on the ground below her second-floor window. She was hypnotized and this child personality was elicited. On formal testing, her visual acuity became 20/60. She could identify people at the back of a large room, which she had been unable to do previously. Furthermore, there was a reduction in her resting nystagmus. When her primary personality re-emerged, her vision reverted to its normal low level. These cases suggest that dissociative processes may activate different control systems that have differing abilities to mobilize optimal visual capacity.

CONCLUSION

Clinical and laboratory research indicates that hypnotic and dissociative states are vehicles for increased control over neurophysiological and peripheral somatic functions. The enhanced ability to modulate perceptual input may facilitate control over output governing respiratory, gastrointestinal, circulatory, and peripheral neural function. This literature suggests that high-hypnotizable individuals and those with dissociative symptoms are capable of an unusual degree of psychological control over various somatic functions, especially those involving parts of the body that are highly visible or available to immediate sensory perception. Much of this control is likely mediated by changes in autonomic nervous system activity as it influences vasodilatation and constriction as well as gastrointestinal activity. Parts of the body that previously experienced physical disease or trauma seem to be especially vulnerable to reactivation of that response with hypnosis. Symptoms compounded by anxiety, such as neurological syndromes and asthma, are likewise susceptible of response to treatment employing hypnosis.

Hypnosis and dissociation thus provide an important opportunity for investigating the limits of psychological control over neurophysiological and somatic processes and for learning more about the relationship between mental state shifts and health.

REFERENCES

Amadeo M, Yanovski A: Evoked potentials and selective attention in subjects capable of hypnotic analgesia. Int J Clin Exp Hypn 23:200–210, 1975

Andreassi JL, Balinsky B, Gallichio JA, et al: Hypnotic suggestion of stimulus change and visual cortical evoked potential. Percept Mot Skills 42:371–378, 1976

Andreychuk T, Skriver C: Hypnosis and biofeedback in the treatment of migraine headache. Int J Clin Exp Hypn 23:172–183, 1975

Apfel RJ, Kelly SF, Frankel FH: The role of hypnotizability in the pathogenesis and treatment of nausea and vomiting of pregnancy. Journal of Psychosomatics and Obstetrics and Gynecology 5:179–186, 1986

Barber TX: Physiological effects of "hypnosis." Psychol Bull 58:390–419, 1961

Baribeau-Braun J, Picton TW, Gosselin JU: A neurophysiological evaluation of abnormal information processing. Science 219:874–876, 1983

Barsky AJ, Wyshak G: Hypochondriasis and somatosensory amplification. Br J Psychiatry 157:404–409, 1990

Beck EC, Barolin GS: The effect of hypnotic suggestion on evoked potentials. J Nerv Ment Dis 140:154–161, 1965

Beck EC, Dustman RD, Beier EG: Hypnotic suggestions and visually evoked potentials. Electroencephalogr Clin Neurophysiol 20:397–400, 1966

Bellis JM: Hypnotic pseudo-sunburn. Am J Clin Hypn 8:310–312, 1966

Bishay EG, Stevens G, Lee C: Hypnotic control of upper gastrointestinal hemorrhage: a case report. Am J Clin Hyp 27:22–25, 1984

Black S: Inhibition of immediate-type hypersensitivity response by direct suggestion under hypnosis. BMJ 1:925–929, 1963a

Black S: Shift in dose-response curve of Prausnitz-Küstner reaction by direct suggestion under hypnosis. BMJ 1:1145–1148, 1963b

Borelli S: Psychische einflusse und reactive haurerscheinungen. Muenchener Medizinische Worhenschelft. 95:1078–1082, 1953

Bramwell JM: Hypnotism: Its History, Practice and Theory. London, Grant Richards, 1903

Chapman LF, Goodell H, Wolff HG. Increased inflammatory reaction induced by central nervous system activity. Trans Assoc Am Physicians 72:84–109, 1959

Clynes M, Kohn M, Lifshitz K: Dynamics and spatial behavior of light-evoked potentials, their modification under hypnosis, and on-line correlation in relation to rhythmic components. Ann N Y Acad Sci 112:468–509, 1964

Colgan SM, Faragher EB, Whorwell PJ: Controlled trial of hypnotherapy in relapse prevention of duodenal ulceration. Lancet 1:1299–1300, 1988

Collison DR: Hypnotherapy in the management of asthma. Am J Clin Hypn 11:6–11, 1968

Collison DR: Which asthmatic patients should be treated by hypnotherapy? Med J Aust 1:776–781, 1975

Davidson RJ, Ekman P, Saron CD, et al: Approach/withdrawal and cerebral asymmetry: emotional expression and brain physiology. J Pers Soc Psychol 58:330–341, 1990

De Pascalis V, Marucci FS, Penna PM: 40-Hz EEG asymmetry during recall of emotional events in waking and hypnosis: differences between low and high hypnotizables. Int J Psychophysiol 7:85–96, 1989

Donchin E, Ritter W, McCallum WC: Cognitive psychophysiology: the endogenous components of the ERP, in Event-Related Brain Potentials in Man. Edited by Callaway E, Tueting P, Koslow SH. New York, Academic Press, 1978, pp 349–411

Dubin LL, Shapiro SS: Use of hypnosis to facilitate dental extraction and hemostasis in a classic hemophiliac with a high antibody titer to factor VIII. Am J Clin Hypn 17:79–83, 1974

Duncan-Johnson CC, Donchin E: The relation of P_{300} latency to reaction time as a function of expectancy. Prog Brain Res 54:717–722, 1980

Edmonston WE, Moscovitz HC: Hypnosis and lateralized brain functions. Int J Clin Exp Hypn 38:70–84, 1990

Esdaile J: Hypnosis in Medicine and Surgery. New York, Julian Press, 1957

Ewin DM: Clinical use of hypnosis for attenuation of burn depth, in Hypnosis at its Bicentennial: Selected Papers. Edited by Frankel FH, Zamansky HS. New York, Plenum, 1978, pp 155–162

Ford JM, Roth WT, Dirk SJ, et al: Evoked potential correlates of signal recognition between and within modalities. Science 181:465–466, 1978

Frankel FH: Significant developments in medical hypnosis during the past 25 years. Int J Clin Exp Hypn 35:231–247, 1987

Frankel FH, Misch RC: Hypnosis in a case of long-standing psoriasis in a person with character problems. Int J Clin Exp Hypn 21:121–130, 1973

Fry L, Mason AA, Bruce-Pearson RS: Effect of hypnosis on allergic skin responses in asthma and hay fever. BMJ 1:1145–1148, 1964

Fung EH, Lazar BS: Hypnosis as an adjunct in the treatment of von Willebrand's disease. Int J Clin Exp Hypn 31:256–265, 1983

Galbraith GC, Cooper LM, London P: Hypnotic susceptibility and the sensory evoked response. Journal of Comparative and Physiological Psychology 80:509–514, 1972

Glaser R, Kiecolt-Glaser J: Stress-associated depression in cellular immunity: implications for acquired immune deficiency syndrome (AIDS). Brain, Behavior, and Immunity 1:107–112, 1987

Glaser R, Kiecolt-Glaser JK, Speicher CE, et al: Stress-related impairments in cellular immunity. Psychiatry Res 16:233–239, 1985

Glaser R, Rice J, Speicher CE, et al: Stress depresses interferon production concomitant with a decrease in natural killer cell activity. Behav Neurosci 100:675–678, 1986

Grabowska MJ: The effect of hypnosis and hypnotic suggestions on the blood flow in the extremities. Polish Medical Journal 10:1044–1051, 1971

Guerrero-Figueroa R, Heath RG: Evoked responses and changes during attentive factors in man. Arch Neurol 10:74–84, 1964

Hadfield JA: The influence of hypnotic suggestion on inflammatory conditions. Lancet 2:678–679, 1917

Halliday AM, Mason AA: Cortical evoked potentials during hypnotic anaesthesia. Electroencephalogr Clin Neurophysiol 16:312–314, 1964

Handford AH, Charney D, Ackerman L, et al: Effect of psychiatric intervention on use of antihemophilic factor concentrate. Am J Psychiatry 137:1254–1256, 1980

Hernandez-Peon R, Donoso M: Influence of attention and suggestion upon subcortical evoked electric activity in the human brain, in First International Congress of Neurological Sciences, Vol 3. Edited by Van Bogaert L, Radermecker J. London, Pergamon, 1959, pp 385–396

Hilgard ER: Divided Consciousness: Multiple Controls in Human Thought and Action. New York, Wiley, 1977

Hilgard ER, Hilgard JR: Hypnosis in the Relief of Pain. Los Altos, CA, William Kaufmann, 1975

Hillyard SA, Picton TW: Sensation, perception, and attention: analysis using ERP's in Event-Related Brain Potentials in Man. Edited by Callaway E, Tueting P, Koslow SH. New York, Academic Press, 1978

Hillyard SA, Picton TW: Event-related brain potentials and selective information processing in man, in Progress in Clinical Neurophysiology, Vol 6. Edited by Desmedt JE. Basel, Switzerland, S Karger, 1979, pp 1–52

Ikemi Y, Nakagawa S: Psychosomatic study of contagious dermatitis. Kyushu Journal of Medical Science 13:335–350, 1962

Johnson R: P$_{300}$ amplitude and probabilistic judgments. Prog Brain Res 54:723–729, 1980

Johnson RFQ, Barber TX: Hypnotic suggestions for blister formation: subjective and physiological effects. Am J Clin Hypn 18:172–181, 1976

Kaneko Z, Takishi N: Psychosomatic studies on chronic urticaria. Folia Psychiatrica Neurologica Japonica 17:16–24, 1963

Kidd CB: Congenital ichthyosiform erythrodermia treated by hypnosis. Br J Dermatol 78:101–105, 1966

Kinsbourne M (ed): Cerebral Hemispheric Function in Depression. Washington, DC, American Psychiatric Press, 1988

Klein KB, Spiegel D: Modulation of gastric acid secretion by hypnosis. Gastroenterology 96:1383–1387, 1989

LeBaron S, Zeltzer L: Research on hypnosis in hemophilia—preliminary success and problems: a brief communication. Int J Clin Exp Hypn 32:290–295, 1984

LeBaw W: Auto-hypnosis in hemophilia. Haematologia 9:103–110, 1975

Locke SE, Ransil BJ, Covino NA, et al: Failure of hypnotic suggestion to alter immune response to delayed-typed hypersensitivity antigens. Ann N Y Acad Sci 496:745–749, 1987

Lubar JF, Gordon DM, Harrist RS, et al: EEG correlates of hypnotic susceptibility based upon fast Fourier power spectral analysis. Biofeedback Self Regul 16:75–85, 1991

Maher-Loughnan GP, Mason AA, MacDonald N, et al: Controlled trial of hypnosis in the symptomatic treatment of asthma. BMJ 2:371–376, 1962

Mason AA: A case of congenital ichthyosiform erythrodermia of brocq treated by hypnosis. BMJ 2:422–423, 1952

Mason AA: Hypnosis and suggestion in the treatment of allergic phenomena. Acta Allergologica 15 (suppl 7):332–338, 1960

Mason AA: Hypnosis and allergy. BMJ 1:1675–1676, 1963

Mishkin M: Cerebral memory circuits, in 1990 Yakult International Symposium: Perception, Cognition and Brain. Tokyo, Japan, Yakult Honsha Co, 1991

Moody RL: Bodily changes during abreaction. Lancet 2:934–935, 1946

Morgan AH, MacDonald H, Hilgard ER: EEG alpha: lateral asymmetry related to task and hypnotizability. Psychophysiology 11:275–282, 1974

Mullins JF, Murray N, Shapiro EM: Pachyonychia congenita: a review and new approach to treatment. Arch Dermatol 17:265–268, 1955

Nemiah JC: Dissociative disorders (hysterical neurosis, dissociative type), in Comprehensive Textbook of Psychiatry, Vol 4. Edited by Kaplan HI, Sadock BJ. Baltimore, MD, Williams & Wilkins, 1985, pp 942–957

Olness K, Culbert T, Uden D: Self-regulation of salivary immunoglobulin A by children. Pediatrics 83:66–71, 1989

Perry C: Imagery, fantasy and hypnotic susceptibility: a multidimensional approach. J Pers Soc Psychol 26:217–221, 1973

Pettinati HM, Wade JH: Hypnosis in the treatment of anorexic and bulimic patients. Seminars in Adolescent Medicine 2:75–79, 1986

Pettinati HM, Horn RL, Staats JS: Hypnotizability in patients with anorexia nervosa and bulimia. Arch Gen Psychiatry 42:1014–1016, 1985

Piccioni C, Hilgard ER, Zimbardo PG: On the degree of stability of measured hypnotizability over a 25-year period. J Pers Soc Psychol 56:289–295, 1989

Posner MI: Chronometric Explorations of Mind. Hillsdale, NJ, Lawrence Erlbaum Associates, 1978

Posner MI, Peterson SE: The attention system of the human brain. Annual Review of Neuroscience 13:25–42, 1990

Posner MI, Klein R, Summers J, et al: On the selection of signals. Memory and Cognition 1:2–12, 1973

Pritchard WS: Psychophysiology of P_{300}. Psychol Bull 89:506–540, 1981

Raynaud JH, Michaex D, Bleirad G, et al: Changes in rectal and mean skin temperature in response to suggested heat during hypnosis in man. Physiol Behav 33:221–226, 1984

Sabourin ME, Cutcomb SD, Crawford HJ, et al: EEG correlates of hypnotic susceptibility and hypnotic trance: spectral analysis and coherence. Int J Psychophysiol 10:125–142, 1990

Sampson RN: Hypnotherapy in a case of pruritus and Guillain-Barré syndrome. Am J Clin Hypn 32:168–173, 1990

Schacter DL: Implicit memory: history and current status. J Exp Psychol Learn Mem Cogn 13:501–518, 1987

Schneck JM: Hypnotherapy for ichthyosis. Psychosomatics 7:233–235, 1966

Serafetinides EA: Electrophysiological responses to sensory stimulation under hypnosis. Am J Psychiatry 125:112–113, 1968

Sheehan PW: Hypnosis and the process of imagination, in Hypnosis Developments in Research and New Perspectives. Edited by Fromm E, Shor RE. New York, Aldine Publishing Company, 1979, pp 381–411

Shor RE, Orne MT, O'Connell DN: Psychological correlates of plateau hypnotizability in a special volunteer sample. J Pers Soc Psychol 4:80–95, 1966

Sigalowitz SJ, Dywan J, Ismailos L: Electrocortical evidence that hypnotically induced hallucinations are experienced. Paper presented at the Society for Clinical and Experimental Hypnosis Meeting as part of a symposium entitled Dissociations in Conscious Experience: Electrophysical and Behavioral Evidence, New Orleans, LA, October 9–13, 1991

Sinclair-Geiben AHC, Chalmers D: Evaluation of treatment of warts by hypnosis. Lancet 2:480–482, 1959

Sjoberg BM, Hollister LE: The effects of psychotomimetic drugs on primary suggestibility. Psychopharmacologia 8:251–262, 1965

Spanos NP: Hypnotic behavior: a social-psychological interpretation of amnesia, analgesia, and "trance logic." Behavioral and Brain Sciences 9:449–502, 1986

Spanos NP: Hypnotic behavior: special process accounts are still not required. Behavioral and Brain Sciences 10:776–781, 1987

Spanos NP, Hewitt EC: The hidden observer in hypnotic analgesia: discovery or experimental creation? J Pers Soc Psychol 39:1201–1204, 1980

Spanos NP, Valois R, Hann MW, et al: Suggestibility and vividness and control of imagery. Int J Clin Exp Hypn 21:305–311, 1973

Spanos MP, Stenstrom RJ, Johnston JC: Hypnosis, placebo, and suggestion in the treatment of warts. Psychosom Med 50:245–260, 1988

Spanos MP, Williams V, Gwynn MI: Effects of hypnotic, placebo, and salicylic acid treatments on wart regression. Psychosocial Medicine 52:109–114, 1990

Spiegel D: Vietnam grief work using hypnosis. Am J Clin Hypn 24:33–40, 1981

Spiegel D: The use of hypnosis in controlling cancer pain. CA Cancer J Clin 35:221–231, 1985; reprinted in Australian Journal of Clinical Hypnotherapy and Hypnosis 7:82–99, 1986

Spiegel D: Seeing through social influence: hypnotic hallucinations are opaque. Behavioral and Brain Sciences 10:775–776, 1987

Spiegel D: Hypnosis, in American Psychiatric Press Textbook of Psychiatry. Edited by Talbott JA, Hales RE, Yudofsy SC. Washington, DC, American Psychiatric Press, 1988, pp 907–928

Spiegel D, Barabasz AF: Effects of hypnotic instructions on P_{300} evoked potential amplitudes: research and clinical implications. Am J Clin Hypn 31:11–17, 1988

Spiegel D, Barbasz A: Psychophysiology of hypnotic hallucination, in Psychophysiology of Mental Imagery: Theory, Research, and Application. Edited by Kunzendorf RG, Sheikh AA. Amityville, NY, Baywood, 1990, pp 133–145

Spiegel D, King R: Hypnotizability and CSF HVA levels among psychiatric patients. Biol Psychiatry 31:95–98, 1992

Spiegel D, Spiegel H: Hypnosis. New York, Basic Books, 1978; reprinted as Trance and Treatment: Clinical Uses of Hypnosis. Washington, DC, American Psychiatric Press, 1987

Spiegel D, Cutcomb S, Ren C, et al: Hypnotic hallucination alters evoked potentials. J Abnorm Psychol 94:249–255, 1985

Spiegel D, Bierre P, Rootenberg J: Hypnotic alteration of somatosensory perception. Am J Psychiatry 146:749–754, 1989

Squires KC, Squires NK, Hillyard SA: Decision-related cortical potentials during an auditory signal detection task with cued observation intervals. J Exp Psychol Hum Percept Perform 1:268–279, 1975

Surman OS, Crumpacker C: Psychological aspects of herpes simplex viral infection: report of six cases. Am J Clin Hypn 30:125–131, 1987

Surman OS, Gottlieb SK, Hackett TP, et al: Hypnosis in the treatment of warts. Arch Gen Psychiatry 28:439–441, 1973

Sutton S, Braren M, Zubin J: Evoked-potential correlates of stimulus uncertainty. Science 150:1187–1188, 1965

Swirsky-Sacchetti T, Margolis CG: The effects of a comprehensive self-hypnosis training program on the use of factor VIII in severe hemophilia. Int J Clin Exp Hypn 34:71–83, 1986

Tellegen A: Practicing the two disciplines for relaxation and enlightenment: comment on "Role of the Feedback Signal in Electromyograph Biofeedback: The Relevance of Attention," by Qualls and Sheegan. J Exp Psychol Gen 110:217–231, 1981

Tellegen A, Atkinson G: Openness to absorbing and self-altering experiences ("absorption"), a trait related to hypnotic susceptibility. J Abnorm Psychol 83:268–277, 1974

Ulich P, Meyer HJ, Biehl B, et al: Cerebral blood flow in autogenic training and hypnosis. Neurosurg Rev 10:P305–P307, 1987

Ullman M: Herpes simplex and second degree burn induced under hypnosis. Am J Psychiatry 103:828–830, 1947

Volkow ND, Tancredi LR: Biological correlates of mental activity studied with PET. Am J Psychiatry 148:439–443, 1991

Wain HJ, Amen D, Jabbari B: The effects of hypnosis on a parkinsonian tremor: case report with polygraph/EEG recordings. Am J Clin Hypn 33:94–98, 1990

Weitzenhoffer AM: Hypnotic susceptibility revisited. Am J Clin Hypn 22:130–146, 1980

Whorwell PJ, Prior A, Faragher EB: Controlled trial of hypnotherapy in the treatment of severe refractory irritable-bowel syndrome. Lancet 1:1232–1234, 1984

Whorwell PJ, Prior A, Colgan SM: Hypnotherapy in severe irritable bowel syndrome: further experience. Gut 28:423–425, 1987

Wilson NJ: Neurophysiologic alterations with hypnosis. Diseases of the Nervous System 29:618–620, 1968

Wilson SC, Barber TX: Vivid fantasy and hallucinatory abilities in the life histories of excellent hypnotic subjects ("somnambules"): preliminary report with female subjects, in Imagery, Vol 2, Concepts, Results, and Applications. Edited by Klinger E. New York, Plenum, 1981, pp 133–149

Wilson SC, Barber TX: The fantasy-prone personality: implication for understanding imagery, hypnosis, and parapsychological phenomena, in Imagery: Current Theory, Research, and Application. Edited by Sheikh AA. New York, Wiley, 1983, pp 340–387

Wink CAS: Congenital ichthyosiform erythrodermia treated by hypnosis: report of two cases. BMJ 2:741–743, 1961

Zachariae R, Bjerring P: The effect of hypnotically induced analgesia on flare reaction of the cutaneous histamine prick test. Arch Dermatol Res 2821:539–543, 1990

Zachariae R, Bjerring P: Increase and decrease of delayed cutaneous reactions obtained by hypnotic suggestions during sensitization: studies on dinitrochlorobenzene and diphenylcyclopropenone. Allergy 48:6–11, 1993

Zachariae R, Bjerring P, Arendt-Nielsen L: Modulation of Type I immediate and Type IV delayed immunoreactivity using direct suggest and guided imagery during hypnosis. Allergy 44:537–542, 1989

Zachariae R, Bjerring P, Arendt-Nielsen L, et al: The effect of hypnotically induced emotional states on brain potentials evoked by painful argon laser stimulation. Clin J Pain 7:130–138, 1991

Zakrzewski K, Szelenberger W: Visual evoked potentials in hypnosis: a longitudinal approach. Int J Clin Exp Hypn 29:77–86, 1981

Zeltzer L, LeBaron S, Zeltzer PM: The effectiveness of behavioral intervention for reduction of nausea and vomiting in children and adolescents receiving chemotherapy. J Clin Oncol 2:683–690, 1984

Zimbardo PG, Maslach C, Marshall G: Hypnosis and the Psychology of Cognitive and Behavioral Control. Stanford, CA, Department of Psychology, Stanford University, 1970

Conclusion

B y now, you have been treated to a variety of approaches to the fascinating phenomenon of dissociation: phenomenological, psychometric, cultural, and psychophysiological. It is hoped that a picture has emerged that is more integrated than dissociated. Although there are many differences among the chapters in this book, there is general agreement that dissociation is fundamental to cognitive function, measurable, sensitive to cultural differences, and important to the mind-body relationship. This suggests a kind of body-mind-body analysis of dissociation. Individuals vary in their capacity to experience dissociation, perhaps due to developmental and biological differences. This means that in any given culture, certain individuals will be more prone than others to experience and express dissociative phenomena. Although certain cultures may teach and encourage the phenomenon more than others, and certain events such as trauma may elicit dissociation, there is additional variance accounted for by differences in individual capacity. Dissociation seems to both arise in response to physical trauma and to be employed in treating the body. Many healing ceremonies overtly elicit or covertly encourage entry into a dissociated state. Dissociation seems to be involved in situations that elicit enhanced psychological control over somatic function, ranging from analgesia to symptom relief of gastrointestinal, neurological, and skin conditions.

PHENOMENOLOGY

It is not strange that dissociation occurs but rather that it does not become evident more often given the general structure of information processing in the brain. The problem may really be the veneer of mental unity we apply to cover the cracks in our complex mental function. It is necessary that various dissociated subunits operate independently, for example, the application of procedural memories that are disentangled from the episodes in which they were learned. Other examples include Professor Erdelyi's work, which shows that repeated recall trials result in enhanced memory. Information that is obviously available, because it emerges on a later recall trial, is kept separate from conscious awareness despite a strenuous effort to elicit it. Furthermore, there may be indirect evidence of its existence via nightmares, fantasies, or the nonrandom results of mere guesses. It is not uncommon for victims of violent crime to be consciously unaware of the details of an assault and yet to have nightmares that present details of it. This perspective makes dissociative phenomena not strange but, if anything, ubiquitous and raises into question our assumption of mental unity.

Indeed, dissociation and hypnosis may represent direct activation of subroutines, either through social or individual input. Hypnotic behavior is relatively automatic and experienced as involuntary. Perhaps hypnosis represents selective and relatively direct access to our procedural memory system. We learn something new (a novel learning episode) but perform it as though it were routine (the result of procedural memory), hence the experience of automaticity in hypnotic and dissociative behavior. Thus dissociation and hypnosis may represent a unique ability to activate mental state, memories, and perceptions without a great deal of processing through consciousness and attention.

These reflections of mine are consistent with the provocative question raised by Professor Bowers: whether dissociation is a consequence of focused attention or whether the obverse may be the case. The narrow boundary of attention may be a consequence of the separation of the mental contents. He uses the observation that a subset of individuals instructed to control pain with hypnosis do better if they simply are told to make it go away. This simple instruction is in contrast to the traditional approach of focusing on an image that implies pain relief, such as warmth or coolness, which for them is less effective. Thus it may be that in a dissociated state, one's focal attention is freed up to do something else. These individuals appear to tap automaticity rather than devote a great deal of central attention to the task of reducing pain hypnotically.

MEASUREMENT

Two excellent instruments for measuring dissociation are presented in this book. One, the Dissociative Experiences Scale, is a continuum measure designed for use in general populations. Higher scores have been shown to typify individuals with histories of physical and sexual abuse and with eating disorders. However, they have not discriminated individuals with pseudoseizures from those without such symptoms. The scale has been successfully translated into several languages and thus applied in several other Western cultures.

The Structured Clinical Interview for DSM-IV Dissociative Disorders is a diagnostic interview schedule that provides considerable precision to the process of obtaining a categorical assessment of a dissociative disorder. It was designed for use among psychiatric patient populations and provides a useful structure of underlying dissociative psychopathology: amnesia, depersonalization, derealization, identity confusion, and identity alteration.

CULTURE AND DISSOCIATION

Trance, dissociation, and hypnosis are overlapping but not identical phenomena. They occur in a variety of Western and non-Western cultures and settings and are powerfully driven by meaning, social interaction, and health significance. Their appearance is influenced by the cultural context in which they are elicited. Hypnosis can be understood as formally induced dissociation, but the ceremonies surrounding it can be understood as heavily influenced by the Western preoccupation with science, rationality, and individuality. The term *induction* arises from Mesmer's discredited theory of animal magnetism, which attempted to bridge science's successful study of influence at a distance (e.g., gravity and magnetism) with his psychotherapeutic approach.

The distinction between subjective and social experience, which is so widely accepted in the West, is of far less importance in Eastern cultures. Thus the clear designation of who is to enter a trance state, typical of Western uses of hypnosis, is less important elsewhere. Non-Western uses of trance often involve music, healing, or religious ceremonies. The notion of *yielding* control of a person's mental state is less alien because the social and intrapsychic worlds are less dichotomized. Trance inductions are more frequently group rather than dyadic events. In particular, the fact that healers often enter trance states as part of healing ceremonies carries with it a suggestion that patients and others observing the ceremony will also enter a trance state. The social setting rather than specific instructions to an individual provides the induction into a trance state.

Cultural norms may have a twofold effect on the nature of dissociative symptoms. They may constitute a likely ground for the expression of symptoms, or they may become a threshold or barrier that raises the severity of stress needed for symptom expression. Dr. Lewis-Fernández points out that possession syndrome is on the one hand more available as a symptom in cultures that have a relatively permeable boundary between self and society. Possession by another identity is not such an alien idea. This makes the syndrome possible, in contrast to cultures that focus more on body integrity, where dissociative symptoms may influence soma more than psyche, for example, in *ataques de nervios*. However, when identity disturbance does occur in Western cultures, the threshold stressors may be higher, as in dissociative identity disorder, which has as precipitants physical and sexual abuse. The higher threshold is the result, in this analysis, of the relative discomfort in the West with the idea of multiple identities. Thus more severe stress is required in Western culture to produce a dissociative identity disturbance, and it is viewed as more abnormal.

It is of great interest to measure hypnosis and dissociation in non-Western cultures, but obstacles include the meaning of Western assessment tools, such as hypnotizability and dissociation scales, in cultures in which trance experience may be considered sacred or in which the examiner's relationship to members of the culture is very important and may influence the result.

PSYCHOPHYSIOLOGY

There are at least three ways in which dissociation, trance, and hypnosis may influence the mind-body relationship:

1. The special relevance of dissociation as a state that in and of itself provides positive health benefits
2. The health-related value of shifts between states (e.g., sleep/wakefulness, trance/nontrance, relaxation/arousal) in maintaining internal homeostasis and/or in buffering the body from the effects of psychological and social stress
3. The use of such altered states with enhanced mental control of physical processes to enact specific strategies resulting in specific effects on specific organ systems

There is at this point little direct evidence that the state itself and shifts among such states positively influence health, although by analogy from the sleep literature this seems plausible. The organism may facilitate internal self-regulation through regular circadian variation. This is more direct evidence that the use of specific attentional efforts in hypnosis has unusual influence on specific organ systems, especially the skin and gastrointestinal system. This is clear evidence of hypnotic effects on the processing of perception in the central nervous system but less clear evidence of effects on clinical pseudoneurological syndromes. Investigations of the effects of hypnosis on the immune system have provided conflicting evidence despite compelling studies of the effects of hypnosis in curing warts, which would seem to implicate an immune effect. This is an exciting area of current research, involving systematic examination of mechanisms by which trance, dissociative, and hypnotic states and/or the contents of them may influence health. Possible pathways include the nervous, circulatory, endocrine, and immune systems. The application of new brain imaging techniques to the problem should yield important answers as will the search for neurotransmitter systems specifically involved in the initiation and maintenance of these mental states.

Although clearly there are difficulties in crossing domains from the cultural through the phenomenological to the neurophysiological and somatic, there seems to be agreement that dissociative phenomena are ubiquitous, that a trait conception of them is useful, and that they often represent extreme and important examples of psychosocial control over somatic processes. Dissociation may not only be better understood through an examination of the influences of culture, mind, and body on the phenomenon, it may also help us better understand the workings of culture, mind, and body.

Index

Index

Index